CASES in HEALTHCARE FINANCE

FOURTH EDITION

LOUIS C. GAPENSKI

In Collaboration with George H. Pink

Health Administration Press, Chicago

Association of University Programs in Health Administration, Arlington, Virginia

Your board, staff, or clients may also benefit from this book's insight. For more information on quantity discounts, contact the Health Administration Press Marketing Manager at (312)424–9470.

This publication is intended to provide accurate and authoritative information in regard to the subject matter covered. It is sold, or otherwise provided, with the understanding that the publisher is not engaged in rendering professional services. If professional advice or other expert assistance is required, the services of a competent professional should be sought.

The statements and opinions contained in this book are strictly those of the author and do not represent the official positions of the American College of Healthcare Executives, the Foundation of the American College of Healthcare Executives, or the Association of University Programs in Health Administration.

Copyright © 2010 by the Foundation of the American College of Healthcare Executives. Printed in the United States of America. All rights reserved. This book or parts thereof may not be reproduced in any form without written permission of the publisher.

15   14   13   12   7   6   5   4

Library of Congress Cataloging-in-Publication Data

Gapenski, Louis C.
  Cases in healthcare finance / Louis C. Gapenski. — 4th ed.
    p. ; cm.
  ISBN 978-1-56793-342-0 (alk. paper)
1. Health facilities—Finance—Case studies. 2. Medical care—Finance—Case studies. I. Title.
  [DNLM: 1. Health Facilities—economics—United States—Case Reports.
2. Health Care Costs—United States—Case Reports. WX 157 G211c 2010]
  RA971.3.G367 2010
  362.1068'1—dc22   2009037787

The paper used in this publication meets the minimum requirements of American National Standard for Information SciencesPermanence of Paper for Printed Library Materials, ANSI Z39.48-19 84.♾™

Acquisitions editor: Janet Davis; Project manager: Jane Calayag; Cover designer: Scott Miller; Layout: BookComp

Found an error or typo? We want to know! Please e-mail it to hap1@ache.org, and put "Book Error" in the subject line.

For photocopying and copyright information, please contact Copyright Clearance Center at www.copyright.com or at (978) 750-8400.

Health Administration Press
A division of the Foundation of the American
    College of Healthcare Executives
One North Franklin Street, Suite 1700
Chicago, IL 60606–3529
(312) 424–2800

Association of University Programs
    in Health Administration
2000 North 14th Street
Suite 780
Arlington, VA 22201
(703) 894–0940

Contents

	Preface for Instructors	ix
	Preface for Students	xix
	Case Descriptions	xxv

Financial Accounting

1	Riverview Community Hospital (A) Assessing Hospital Performance	3
2	Chesapeake Health Plans Assessing HMO Performance	15

Managerial Accounting

3	Rio Grande Medical Center Cost Allocation Concepts	27
4	Apple Valley Family Practice Cost Allocation Methods	35
5	Blue Pointe Healthcare Premium Development	41
6	Columbia Memorial Hospital Break-even Analysis	49
7	Palisades Mental Health Clinic Variance Analysis	55
8	Alpine Village Clinic Cash Budgeting	65
9	Boston Transplant Center Marginal Cost Pricing Analysis	71
10	Denver Health Network ABC Analysis	77
11	Maitland Family Physicians Pay for Performance	83

Financial Management Basics

12	Pensacola Surgery Centers Time Value Analysis	95
13	Southeastern Specialty, Inc. Financial Risk	101
14	Atlantic Healthcare (A) Bond Valuation	107
15	Atlantic Healthcare (B) Stock Valuation	113

Capital Acquisition

16	Southern Homecare Cost of Capital	121
17	RN Temp Services, Inc. Capital Structure Analysis	127
18	Portland Cancer Center Leasing Decisions	135

Capital Investment

19	Palms Hospital Traditional Project Analysis	143
20	American Rehabilitation Centers Staged Entry Analysis	149
21	Cook County Health System Make or Buy Analysis	155
22	St. Jerome Teaching Hospital Merger Analysis	163
23	South Beach Health Partners Joint Venture Analysis	171
24	Bloomington Clinics Practice Valuation	181
25	University Faculty Practice Physician Extender Analysis	187
26	Johnson Memorial Hospital Competing Technologies with Backfill	193

Working Capital

27	Commonwealth Pharmaceuticals Receivables Management	201
28	Clear Lake Hospital Inventory Management	207

Other Topics

29	Riverview Community Hospital (B) Financial Forecasting	215
30	Copperline Healthcare Capitation and Risk Sharing	219

Ethics Mini-Cases

1	Trigon Blue Cross/Blue Shield Copayments	227
2	Deal of a Lifetime Corporate-Owned Life Insurance	229
3	Bayview Surgery Center Pricing/Billing of Surgical Services	231
4	Jefferson General Hospital Mergers, Acquisitions, and Agency	233
5	Front Street Hospital Uninsured Charges and Collections	235
6	Westwood Imaging Centers Payment for Referrals	239

About the Author	243
About the Contributor	245

Preface for Instructors

HEALTHCARE FINANCE CAN be a fascinating, exciting subject, yet students often regard it as either too theoretical or too mechanical. The fact is good financial decision making requires both good theory and good quantitative work plus a great deal of insight and judgment. The best way to get this point across to students, and to demonstrate the inherent richness of the subject matter, is to relate classroom work to real-world decision making. When this is done, students must not only grapple with the concepts but, more important, with how the concepts are applied in practice.

Of course, the most realistic application of healthcare finance occurs within healthcare organizations, and there is no substitute for "on-the-job" experience. The next best thing, and the only real option for the classroom, is to use cases to simulate the environment in which financial decisions are actually made. The purpose of this casebook is to provide students with an opportunity to bridge the gap between learning concepts in a classroom setting and actually applying them on the job. By using these cases, students can be better prepared to deal with the multitude of problems that arise in the practice of healthcare finance.

Content

This casebook primarily consists of 30 cases that focus on the practice of healthcare finance within various types of healthcare organizations. In general, each case addresses a single financial issue, such as a capital investment decision, but the uncertainty of the input data, along with the presence of relevant nonfinancial factors, makes each case interesting and challenging. Because the cases focus on both accounting and financial management decisions, they cover the full range of healthcare finance. Furthermore, the case settings include a wide variety of organizational settings, including hospitals, clinics, medical practices, home health care organizations, integrated delivery systems, and managed care organizations.

In addition to healthcare finance cases, the casebook contains six ethics mini-cases. Each mini-case contains a very short description of a finance situation that has potential ethical implications. These cases require no numerical analysis; rather, they are intended to be used as discussion vehicles for instructors who want to include finance-related ethics content in their healthcare finance courses.

Changes in the Fourth Edition

I have used the third edition in more than ten courses since its publication. Moreover, I have received comments and suggestions from numerous users in different settings. This feedback has resulted in many changes; a few are substantial and a great deal are minor.

The most substantial change to the casebook involves authorship. This edition was written in collaboration with George H. Pink, a professor of health policy and management at the University of North Carolina at Chapel Hill. As you may know, George also is joining me as coauthor on *Understanding Healthcare Financial Management*, the book that is often used as a reference text with the casebook. George brings new insights to the cases that, beginning with this edition, will have a profound and positive impact on the book.

A few of the cases have had major revisions:

- **Case 9 (Boston Transplant Center):** This marginal cost pricing analysis case has been expanded to include both underlying cost structure and current profitability information. Thus, students can apply total cost and profitability analysis on top of marginal cost and profitability. The case also encourages students to consider long-term and short-term implications.

- **Case 11 (Maitland Family Physicians):** This pay-for-performance (P4P) case has been expanded to include three areas of performance (productivity, finance, and quality), whereas the previous version focused almost exclusively on financial performance. Students can select from among nine performance measures, each of which has different strengths and limitations. The case better illustrates the incentives, data burden, internal politics, and difficulties involved in implementing a P4P plan.
- **Case 24 (Bloomington Clinics):** This clinic valuation case has been expanded to include the use of free operating cash flow as a valuation approach in addition to valuations based on free cash flow to equityholders, number of physicians, and revenues. Also, debt financing has been added to the clinic's capital structure, which increases the complexity of the financial statements and valuation analyses.
- **Chapter 27 (Commonwealth Pharmaceuticals):** This receivables management case has been modified to make it more realistic. The firm now has four customers instead of two, and each customer has a different receivables collection pattern. The greater number of customers makes interpretation of changes in the accounts receivables balances, average collection period, aging schedule, and uncollected balances schedule more complicated. In addition, the cost of carrying receivables has been added to the model, which permits analyses of the trade-offs between the costs and benefits of actions taken to reduce receivables balances.
- **Case 30 (Copperline Healthcare):** This capitation and risk-sharing case has been recast as a new Physician Hospital Organization (PHO) that must decide (1) how to allocate the premium dollars collected from its first contract to its different classes of providers and (2) what reimbursement methods it should use. The premium allocation has been expanded to include more provider components, which requires students to consider more factors when making the revenue

allocation decision. In addition, the case model now includes sensitivity analyses to assess how changes in allocations from the professional services and inpatient services risk pools are affected by changes in the premium allocation.

In addition to these major revisions, many smaller changes have been made to improve both the cases and the spreadsheet models. Regarding the cases, all case titles were changed, and numerous alterations were made to the case settings and numerical values to make the cases more beneficial for students. Regarding the models, many changes, mostly minor, were made to make the models easier to understand and use as well as more valuable to the case analyses.

Our primary goal in making these changes was to improve the pedagogic value of the cases. In addition, in cases without major changes, we modified a number or two to change the solutions slightly, ensuring that the new edition presents a fresh challenge to students. Still, we did not want to change the underlying character of the cases because (1) they work well now and (2) we do not want instructors to have to relearn the cases each time a new edition is published.

Directed Versus Nondirected Cases

In general, cases may be classified as directed or nondirected. Directed cases include a specific set of questions that students must answer to complete the case, while nondirected cases (as we use the term) contain only general guidance to point students in the right direction. Most of the cases in this book are nondirected. (Cases 12 through 15, which focus on basic finance concepts rather than applications, are directed.) The primary advantage of nondirected cases is that they closely resemble how real-world managers confront financial decision making because they require students to develop their own solution approach. The disadvantage is that students who stray from the key issues of the case often do not obtain full value from their effort.

In general, students with more advanced analytical and logic skills gain the most from nondirected cases, while students who have had less exposure to casework gain the most from directed cases. The online Instructor's Resources contains a set of questions for each nondirected case that can be used to convert the nondirected into directed cases. Thus, instructors have the option of using the cases in either way, depending on the experience of the students, the objectives of the course, and the extent to which the cases will be used.

Use of This Casebook

The cases in this book can be used in several different ways. For example, these cases form the foundation for the second healthcare finance course in the University of Florida's MHA program. Students in this program take an introductory healthcare finance course that includes both accounting and financial management basics, so the second course focuses on the **application** of finance concepts within healthcare organizations. The course is essentially a pure case course, and about 15 cases (one per week) are assigned. The students have had sufficient lecture work in healthcare finance, so at this stage learning by doing is most important. The students are not provided with the accompanying case questions, so they must develop their own approaches to completing each case.

A group of three to four students is assigned to present each assigned case in class. Group work is an excellent experience for students because almost all decision making in businesses is done in a group environment, and people who cannot work in groups are doomed to failure. Students will need to know how to motivate people who work for them, and students will need to be able to work with others in a cooperative manner.

Many students wish that they did not have to work in groups because doing their own thing at their own convenience is much easier. Because the world does not work that way, learning to work with others is better done now while mistakes are less costly. Typically, the highest-quality case analyses are conducted by cooperative teams that discuss the issues and methods. Generally, some team members will be good at spreadsheet modeling, others will be good writers or good with word processing or presentation software, while others will be good at identifying and analyzing the relevant points in the cases. By combining those talents, the group can produce a better analysis and presentation than can one student working individually.

An in-class group presentation of the cases also provides students the opportunity to hone their presentation skills, including the use of presentation software such as Microsoft PowerPoint. Healthcare executives constantly state that the ability to communicate is absolutely critical to success in business. We agree completely. A knowledge of healthcare finance (or any other managerial discipline) is useless unless the individual can communicate his or her ideas to others. Students who are not presenting the case must work the case individually (or perhaps in groups) and then act as members of the board of directors during the presentation. They are responsible for asking relevant questions of the presenting group and pointing out any deficiencies in the analysis.

In addition to use in a pure case course, the cases can also be used in other ways. For example, the MHA program at the University of North Carolina at Chapel Hill has two second-year healthcare finance courses. The first course covers basic financial management concepts, capital acquisition, cost of capital, and capital structure. The second course covers capital allocation, financial condition analysis and forecasting, and other topics. Each course includes six to seven cases, which the students either present or discuss in class as guided by the instructor.

Finally, we find that the cases work particularly well in Executive MHA programs. Executive students generally bring a great deal of real-world insights into their case analyses, which results in lively discussions. In addition, the cases can be worked during the intervals between on-campus sessions, which allows plenty of time for group discussion and analysis.

Spreadsheet Models

Spreadsheet analysis has become extremely important in all aspects of healthcare finance. Students should be given the opportunity to develop computer skills and be allowed, or required, to use spreadsheet programs to assist in case analyses. If students have not previously used spreadsheets, they must be exposed to them because functional literacy in any area of management today requires a knowledge of spreadsheet modeling. Furthermore, spreadsheet models can reduce the amount of busywork required to perform the calculations and hence leave students with more time to focus on finance issues.

Because of these factors, we developed well-structured, user-friendly spreadsheet models for all cases except those that focus on building skills as opposed to applying them. The spreadsheet models are efficient and hence big time savers, especially when conducting risk assessment using techniques such as sensitivity and scenario analyses. In addition, spreadsheet models allow students to easily create graphics and other computer output that enhance the quality of both analyses and presentations.

Spreadsheet models are available for 26 of the 30 cases. Those cases without models focus on basic principles that underlie mathematical calculations (Cases 12–15, the financial management basics cases). The best way for students to learn these principles is to perform the calculations from scratch, using either a calculator or a spreadsheet program to ease the burden.

In thinking about student use of these models, an important question arose: Should we provide complete models to the students, or should students be required to do some (or all) of the modeling themselves? After using several different approaches, we concluded that the best solution is to provide students with complete versions of the case models in the sense that no modeling is required to obtain a base case solution. However, zeros have been entered for all input data in the student versions, and hence students must identify and then enter the appropriate input data. When this is done, the model automatically calculates the base case solution. However, the models do not contain risk analyses or other extensions such as graphics, so students must modify the models as necessary to make them most useful in completing the cases. The student versions of the case models can be downloaded from the Health Administration Press website at www.ache.org/books/FinanceCases4.

The instructor versions of the case models are similar to the student versions, except that the input values are intact. Thus, instructors can view the base case solution without entering any data. In addition, some instructor-version models include additional modeling, such as risk analyses.

Instructor's Resources

Several teaching aids are available for instructors who adopt this book. Contact hap1@ache.org to gain access to these files.

- *PowerPoint slides.* The essential material needed for each case is summarized in a set of introductory slides. Instructors may use these slides if students need

an in-class review. Hard-copy versions (or the files themselves) may be provided to students if desired. Instructors may either use the slides "as is" or customize them to meet the needs of the class.
- *Case questions.* A set of questions for each case is available for instructors who want to convert the cases from nondirected to directed.
- *Case solutions.* Each case has a comprehensive solution based on the case questions.
- *Instructor models.* The instructor's version of the spreadsheet models may be downloaded.

Acknowledgments

This casebook reflects the efforts of many people. First, George Pink created many improvements along the way. On several of the cases, he was ably assisted by Robert Harmon, a student in the University of North Carolina's Department of Health Policy and Management.

Also, four of the cases were coauthored by the following colleagues at the University of Florida or at Shands Healthcare, an affiliate of the University of Florida:

- Murray Côté
- Ian Jamieson
- Brett Justice
- Paul Phillips

Finally, colleagues, students, and staff at the University of Florida provided inspirational support, as well as more tangible support, during the development and class testing of the revised cases. In addition, the Health Administration Press staff was instrumental in ensuring the quality and usefulness of this casebook.

Conclusion

The field of healthcare finance continues to undergo significant changes and advances. Participating in these developments is stimulating, and we sincerely hope that the fourth edition of *Cases in Healthcare Finance* will help students gain a better appreciation for the application of finance principles to healthcare organizations.

A book that raises so many issues will also inevitably generate a variety of opinions regarding financial theory and practice. Furthermore, although both the publisher and I have placed great emphasis on the accuracy of the cases, some discrepancies or inconsistencies may exist. We would appreciate any comments, corrections, criticisms, and ideas for improving all aspects of the cases and related materials. Also, if any technical problems arise with the models, feel free to contact me directly.

Professor Louis C. Gapenski, PhD
Department of Health Services Research, Management and Policy
Box 100195, Health Science Center
University of Florida
Gainesville, FL 32610–0195
E-mail: gapenski@ufl.edu

Preface for Students

THERE IS NO better way to learn healthcare finance than by working cases. Of course, first, it is necessary to have a basic understanding of the principles and concepts that will be applied in the cases, and this knowledge generally is obtained from previous work.

The primary emphasis of the finance cases in this book is to present situations that require analysis and judgment regarding financial decision making. Although the emphasis here is on financial analysis, real-world decisions are based as much (perhaps more) on qualitative factors as on numbers. This means that it is important that you consider not only the financial implications of the cases but also the relevant nonfinancial considerations before reaching final conclusions and making recommendations.

As you work these cases, recognize that in most situations there is more than one right answer. Indeed, in some cases, multiple approaches to the solution may be appropriate. The critical issue in presenting your findings is supporting your conclusions and recommendations. Note that the guidance given here is generic in nature and does not take precedence over the guidance provided by your instructor.

Obtaining the Case Spreadsheet Models

All finance cases, except the financial management basics cases (12–15), have accompanying spreadsheet models. These models can be downloaded from the Health Administration Press website at www.ache.org/

books/FinanceCases4. Note that the input data in these models have been zeroed out. Thus, you will have to enter the appropriate values for these data to get the models to "work." Also, note that the models contain only base case analyses. You must add to the models any extensions required by the case, such as risk analyses and graphics (charts).

Working a Case

Of course, there is an unlimited number of approaches to working the cases, and the approach that is optimal for one individual (or group) is not necessarily the best for another individual (or group). That said, here are suggested steps to help in your casework. (Note that the cases differ in content, and hence one size [the steps below] does not fit all.)

1. Scan the case to get an overall idea of the setting, topic, and decision at hand.
2. Look at the accompanying spreadsheet model to get a feel for its structure and the nature of the input data needed.
3. Read the case to identify alternative courses of action and to extract the data needed (typically model inputs) for the numerical analysis.
4. Enter the base case data into the spreadsheet model, and check for any problems that might arise, including illogical results.
5. Conduct scenario, sensitivity, and other analyses as needed to either assess risk or make judgments about how uncertainty affects alternative courses of action.
6. Identify the qualitative factors that bear on the decision at hand. Don't forget this one!
7. Reach your final conclusions, which should logically lead to your recommendations.

Most of the information required to successfully work a case is contained in the case itself. However, you may encounter situations in which additional information would allow you either to feel more comfortable in your recommendations or to examine out-of-the-box solutions. By all means, feel free to pull data from other sources as needed to create a more complete case solution. In fact, if the data needed are not easily available from other sources, there is nothing wrong with making your own assumptions, as long as they pass the "reasonableness" test.

Making a Presentation

Many of you will be required to present your case analysis in class, either as individuals or as a group. Generally, your audience will not have written material to refer to (except for supporting financial statements, numerical tables, and so on). Thus, you must structure your presentation so that it can be easily followed and understood the first time around. Although most cases involve a great deal of detailed information, your presentation will be easy to follow if it is simply and clearly organized.

All effective presentations consist of three parts: (1) an introduction, (2) a body (analysis), and (3) conclusions and recommendations. The first step in preparing a presentation is to construct the body. This is the analysis that must convince the audience that your conclusions and recommendations have merit. If the body is too long and complex, the audience will not be able to grasp its implications and hence will not understand the rationale behind your conclusions and recommendations. Conversely, an analysis that is too short will appear to be lacking in thought and substance and will raise more questions than answers. Similarly, a body that is not presented in a step-wise, logical sequence may contain the right information but still not get the job done because the audience just can't follow its logic.

Once the body of the presentation has been prepared, the introduction and conclusions and recommendations should be added. The introduction serves three purposes: (1) to gain the audience's attention, (2) to describe the decision at hand, and (3) to present the main ideas that will be covered in the remainder of the presentation.

A presentation can have an excellent introduction and body, but it may still be totally ineffective. There is nothing worse than a presentation that trails off "into the sunset," leaving the audience wondering why they just spent 30 minutes listening. The conclusions and recommendations must be strong and convincing so that the audience knows that a sound and thorough analysis has been accomplished. In essence, the conclusions and recommendations should provide closure for the audience. Any questions remaining at this point should involve technical details as opposed to "What did you say we should do?"

Preparing the Slides

In most cases, you will be using PowerPoint slides as the basis for the presentations. Don't forget that the primary function of slides is to support your message. Thus, the slides must contain the key elements of the introduction, body (analysis), and conclusions and recommendations. Slides that are irrelevant or confusing detract from the presentation. Also, too many slides is just as confusing to the audience as too few slides.

Don't try to put a great deal of numerical detail on slides. For example, several years of financial statements on a single slide will not be readable from the back of the room. Similarly, breaking the statements into sections so that they are on multiple slides is also a poor idea because the audience will not be able to see all the data at one time. For large amounts of data, handouts are preferable to slides. The key points should be on slides, but use handouts to provide the audience with numerical details.

Working in Groups

There is a good chance that you will be working in groups. For many students, group work is a blessing; for others, it is a curse. The advantage of working in groups is that more talent typically is brought to the table. The disadvantage is that group work can create logistical problems, such as When can the group meet? and What is each group member's role?

Good groups recognize comparative advantage and capitalize on it. Students who are good at spreadsheets can be the "geeks," students who are good at problem solving can be the "brains," students who are good slide makers can be the "artists," and students who are good at verbal communications can be the "faces." There is nothing wrong with focusing on individuals' strengths. However, each member of the group is still accountable for all phases of the work. All group members must actively review and approve the work done by other team members. If one member of the group makes a major error, this fact must be noted and corrected by the other members of the group. If a group allows one member to sink the ship, then the entire group is going to drown. Groups in which individuals play different roles do the best casework, but all members ultimately review and approve the final product.

Some Final Words

When all is said and done, the key to a good case analysis and presentation is preparedness: Proper prior planning prevents poor performance. This philosophy applies to all phases of casework, including the presentation itself. How many times have you witnessed a presentation that starts 15 minutes late because the laptop or projector doesn't work or one of the presenters is late? Or, midway through the presentation, a slide either is missing or contains typographical errors? Such events can easily be, and should be, prevented by proper planning. Such "small things" cast a shadow of doubt over the analysis and presentation and hence reflect poorly on the entire effort.

Professor Louis C. Gapenski, PhD
Department of Health Services Research, Management and Policy
Box 100195, Health Science Center
University of Florida
Gainesville, FL 32610–0195
E-mail: gapenski@ufl.edu

Case Descriptions

Case 1: This case discusses the financial statement analysis of a 210-bed hospital. It requires EVA (economic value added) analysis, Du Pont analysis, financial ratio analysis, and operating ratio analysis. The case has an accompanying spreadsheet model that contains five years of historical data, industry average data, and a complete calculation of relevant ratios and Du Pont analysis.

Case 2: This case is similar to Case 1, except it focuses on the managed care industry. It presents two years of data and discusses benchmarking against primary competitors as well as the industry; thus, here, the analysis and interpretation are somewhat different from those in Case 1.

Case 3: This case focuses on the question, What constitutes a good cost driver? Here, students must ponder the "fairness" of allocating a higher amount of facilities overhead to a department that is being forced to move to a new facility. The case raises other issues regarding cost drivers, fairness, and cost-reduction effectiveness.

Case 4: This case focuses on the mechanics of cost allocation. It asks students to use four allocation methods (direct, step down, double apportionment, and reciprocal) to allocate costs from three support departments to three patient service departments.

Case 5: This case focuses on the development of a premium rate to be offered to a buyer consortium. Here, students must deal with coverage limitations and copays, as well as the basic costs of providing services, when developing the premium rate.

Case 6: This case involves the break-even analysis of an unprofitable walk-in clinic owned by a hospital. Because the spreadsheet model for this case does the busywork, students can concentrate on the problems inherent in break-even analysis and its value to managers in making service decisions.

Case 7: This case focuses on the budget variance analysis of four managed care product lines. Because of the nature of variance analysis, the accompanying spreadsheet model handles the required calculations. To add to the mathematical complexity, the case involves both utilization and enrollment differences.

Case 8: This case is a traditional cash budgeting exercise. It calls for students to develop six monthly budgets as well as a daily budget for a single month. The spreadsheet model, which reduces the amount of busywork required, facilitates sensitivity analyses regarding both patient volume and collection experience. The case presents students with an opportunity to discuss many facets of cash management.

Case 9: This case focuses on the pricing of transplant services. It requires students to do some calculations but does not require a large-scale quantitative effort. The primary purpose of the case is to allow students to consider alternative (full versus marginal) cost definitions when pricing a service.

Case 10: This case focuses on using ABC (activity-based costing) techniques to estimate the costs associated with two alternative approaches to providing ultrasound services. The accompanying spreadsheet model takes out much of the busywork. The case calls for sensitivity analysis on many input variables and consideration of various qualitative factors that affect the selection decision.

Case 11: This case involves the measurement of physician productivity, financial performance, and quality of care and its use in determining pay for performance. Alternative methodologies are proposed in the case, and students must choose among those given. The case also raises issues about how compensation systems should be trusted, understood, equitable, and affordable and should provide proper incentives.

Case 12: This case focuses on the mechanics of time value analysis. Because the case is meant to make students think about the time value process, it does not have an accompanying spreadsheet model. The case contains a set of questions that lead students through the case. The question format is best applied to cases that focus on fundamental concepts rather than managerial decision making.

Case 13: This case focuses on basic financial risk concepts. Its goal is to give students a sound understanding of the three types of financial risk (stand-alone, corporate, and market) and their implications for decision making within healthcare organizations. Like Case 12, the case contains a set of questions that lead students through the required concepts and has no accompanying spreadsheet model.

Case 14: This case focuses on the mechanics of bond valuation as opposed to the managerial decisions inherent in floating a bond issue. This case has no accompanying spreadsheet model and contains a set of questions that students must answer. Here, much of the bond valuation work is at a basic level, but the case includes questions pertaining to yield to call and expected rate of return when an issue has a sinking fund.

Case 15: This case takes students through the mechanics of stock valuation (not the managerial decision process that surrounds a new stock issue), including both the constant and nonconstant growth dividend models. No spreadsheet model is included, and the case contains a set of questions that students must answer.

Case 16: This case focuses on the estimation of a business's cost of capital, including both corporate and divisional costs. Because the required calculations are relatively simple, the accompanying spreadsheet model is very basic. However, students have to grapple with numerous conceptual issues regarding both estimation methodologies and the interpretation and use of the cost of capital once it is estimated.

Case 17: This case examines the capital structure decision for an investor-owned company that franchises "rent-a-nurse" businesses. Here, the primary analytical tool is a zero-growth model that calculates stock price under alternative capital structures. However, the case also examines the impact of financial leverage on accounting profits and asks students to consider the business's value under two theoretical models (Modigliani-Miller and Miller). Also, the case requires students to consider qualitative factors in making the final decision. The accompanying spreadsheet model eases the mathematical busywork.

Case 18: This case looks at the equipment leasing decision facing a hospital. The case requires students to perform both lessee's and lessor's analyses. The case brings out many side issues, including the correct discount rate, dealing with residual value uncertainty, the impact of cancellation and per procedure clauses, and the effects on both parties of leveraging the lease. To ease calculations, the case has an accompanying spreadsheet model.

Case 19: This case contains a traditional (no twists) capital budgeting analysis, including cash flow estimation, decision measures, risk assessment, and risk incorporation. In evaluating the financial attractiveness of a proposed outpatient surgery center, students are confronted with many of the problems that occur in such analyses. An accompanying spreadsheet model helps with the calculations. This is a good case for illustrating Monte Carlo simulation.

Case 20: This case focuses on the advantages of making significant capital investments in stages rather than one large investment at a single point in time. In particular, the case uses a decision tree methodology to determine project risk and to illustrate the benefits of abandonment. The accompanying spreadsheet model permits students to spend more time on concepts rather than on number crunching and takes the tedium out of the calculations.

Case 21: This case investigates several alternative proposals for a hospital system's print shop, including closing the shop and outsourcing. The case includes a spreadsheet model and discusses several technical issues related to discounted cash flow analysis, such as the handling of non-normal cash flows. Finally, the case examines the strategic issue of entering the for-profit printing market.

Case 22: This case explores the valuation of a not-for-profit hospital for possible acquisition by another not-for-profit hospital. In addition to the numerical analysis, the case raises several issues related to control after the merger. The accompanying spreadsheet model does the busywork, but students must think a great deal about the impact of the merger on both entities and how future cash flows will be affected.

Case 23: This case focuses on the analysis of a proposed joint venture involving three equity partners: a hospital and group practice (the general partners) and individual physicians (the limited partners). Here, students must consider both the costs of capital for the partners and how the partnership cash flows should be allocated across the equity participants. The case addresses several qualitative issues, including the risks associated with new, unproven technology and the ethical (and legal) issues involved in income-generating referrals. The spreadsheet model does most of the numerical work.

Case 24: This case requires students to value a family physician group practice. The case provides data to allow students to use both DCF (discounted cash flow) and market multiple methodologies. Because of a host of both qualitative and quantitative issues, the ultimate "answer" here is filled with uncertainties. More data are given in this case than in Case 22, so fewer assumptions are required. The spreadsheet model helps with the calculations.

Case 25: This case focuses on the financial assessment of the use of physician extenders in three clinical settings. Here, students must make judgments about whether a physician assistant or a nurse practitioner is better suited for particular types of clinic operations. The spreadsheet model eases the quantitative burden, but the real work is in making the hard assumptions needed to deal with extender impact on volume, reimbursement, and costs.

Case 26: This case focuses on a capital investment decision that involves the use of alternative technologies. To complicate the analysis, one technology frees up inpatient beds for alternative purposes (backfill). The case examines a simplistic replacement analysis, which also makes students consider the differences in replacement versus new project analyses. The accompanying spreadsheet model facilitates the calculations.

Case 27: This case focuses on the basics of receivables management. A start-up drug company is used to illustrate such concepts as average collection period (ACP, also known as DSO or days sales outstanding), aging schedules, uncollected balances schedules, and the cost of carrying receivables. To complicate matters, these concepts must be applied to multiple customers.

Case 28: This case leads students through an inventory decision process involving supplier selection and optimal ordering quantity (and hence inventory level). The case focuses primarily on the economic ordering quantity model, although students must also categorize inventory items according to the ABC model. The accompanying spreadsheet model facilitates the calculations.

Case 29: This case, which builds on the information given in Case 1, focuses on the development of a set of forecasted financial statements for the hospital. It encompasses both forecasting and financial accounting considerations. The accompanying spreadsheet model provides a framework for the forecasting process. However, students must modify the model to incorporate more appropriate forecasting techniques and more realistic operating assumptions. This case requires students to make an extensive set of assumptions about both the future of the hospital industry and one particular hospital.

Case 30: This case focuses on the problems faced by a PHO (physician-hospital organization) when one of its most important payers proposes a fixed per member per month payment. This situation forces the PHO to consider how to handle a full-risk contract related to both utilization risk and how the fixed payment and the associated risk should be shared among the hospital, specialist physicians, and primary care physicians. The accompanying spreadsheet model makes it easier for students to assess the impact of their assumptions.

Mini-Cases

Ethics Case 1: This case discusses a situation in which a patient pays a copayment based on full charges while the insurer pays much less than full charges because of contractual discounts.

Ethics Case 2: This case explores the issues associated with corporate ownership (in which the corporation is the beneficiary) of individual life insurance policies.

Ethics Case 3: This case is the flip side of Ethics Case 1. Here, a lower price (and copayment) is quoted to the patient while the insurer pays a higher amount.

Ethics Case 4: This case focuses on the personal conflicts that arise when the CEO of a small, not-for-profit hospital is confronted with multiple takeover bids.

Ethics Case 5: This case discusses the dilemma that hospitals face in treating the uninsured. How much should hospitals charge the uninsured for services provided, and how aggressive should they be in pursuing those collections?

Ethics Case 6: This case centers on the financial arrangements being used by some imaging services companies to "encourage" physicians to refer patients to their centers. Are these arrangements legal? If so, are the arrangements ethical?

The following case is available only online at www.ache.org/books/FinanceCases4

Waverly Enterprises: This case focuses on the mechanics of the bond refunding decision. The case raises several qualitative issues and poses a situation where the maturity of the new issue exceeds the remaining life of the issue to be refunded. The accompanying spreadsheet model assumes annual coupons, giving students a chance to demonstrate their modeling skills by requiring them to modify the model to accommodate semiannual coupons.

*Financial
Accounting*

RIVERVIEW COMMUNITY HOSPITAL (A)
ASSESSING HOSPITAL PERFORMANCE

RIVERVIEW COMMUNITY HOSPITAL is a 210-bed, not-for-profit, acute care hospital with a long-standing reputation for providing quality healthcare services to a growing service area. Riverview competes with three other hospitals in its metropolitan statistical area (MSA)—two not-for-profit and one for-profit. It is the smallest of the four but has traditionally been ranked highest in patient satisfaction polls.

Hospitals are accredited by the Joint Commission, an independent not-for-profit organization whose mission is to improve the safety and quality of healthcare provided to the public through accreditation and related services. (For more information on the Joint Commission, visit their website at www.jointcommission.org.) Although accreditation is optional for hospitals, it is generally required to qualify for governmental (Medicare and Medicaid) reimbursement, and hence the vast majority of hospitals apply for accreditation. Riverview passed its latest Joint Commission accreditation with "flying colors," receiving full accreditation, the highest of the accreditation categories.

In recent years, competition among the four hospitals in Riverview's service area has been keen but friendly. However, a large for-profit chain recently purchased the for-profit hospital, which has resulted in some anxiety among the managers of the other three hospitals because of the chain's reputation for aggressively increasing market share in the markets they serve.

Relevant financial and operating data for Riverview are contained in Exhibits 1.1 through 1.4, and selected industry data are contained in

4   *Cases in Healthcare Finance*

Exhibits 1.5 and 1.6. (Note that the industry data given in the case are for illustrative purposes only and do not represent actual data for the years specified. For a better idea of the type of comparative data actually available for hospitals, see the Ingenix website at www.hospitalbenchmarks.com.)

In addition to the data in the exhibits, the following information was extracted from the notes section of Riverview's 2009 Annual Report.

1. A significant portion of the hospital's net patient service revenue was generated by patients who are covered by either Medicare, Medicaid, or other government programs or by various private plans, including managed care plans, that have contracts with the hospital that specify discounts from charges. In general, the proportional amount of deductions is similar between inpatients and outpatients. The gross/net revenue breakdown for both inpatient and outpatient services is as follows (in millions of dollars):

	2005	2006	2007	2008	2009
Gross patient service revenue					
Inpatient	$25.161	$25.275	$26.117	$29.148	$33.216
Outpatient	4.748	5.969	6.535	9.130	11.912
Gross patient revenue	$29.909	$31.244	$32.652	$38.278	$45.128
Revenue deductions					
Contractual allowances	$ 2.489	$ 2.053	$ 1.729	$ 5.196	$ 7.516
Charity care	1.759	1.955	2.127	2.506	3.030
Total deductions	$ 4.248	$ 4.008	$ 3.856	$ 7.702	$10.546
Net patient service revenue	$25.661	$27.236	$28.796	$30.576	$34.582

2. Inventories are stated at the lower of costs—determined on a first-in, first-out basis—or market value.
3. The breakdown of operating expenses between inpatient and outpatient activities is as follows (in millions of dollars):

	2005	2006	2007	2008	2009
Inpatient expenses	$18.635	$19.221	$20.573	$22.229	$24.771
Outpatient expenses	5.261	6.062	6.831	8.098	9.187
Total operating expenses	$23.896	$25.283	$27.404	$30.327	$33.958

4. Riverview has a contributory money accumulation (defined contribution) pension plan that covers substantially all of its employees. Participants can contribute up to 20 percent of earnings to the pension plan. The hospital matches, on a dollar-for-dollar basis, employee contributions of up to 2 percent of wages and pays 50 cents on the dollar for contributions of more than 2 percent and up to 4 percent. Because the plan is a defined contribution plan (as opposed to a defined benefit plan), there are no unfunded pension liabilities. Pension expense was approximately $0.543 million in 2008 and $0.588 million in 2009.

5. The hospital is a member of the State Hospital Trust Fund under which it purchases professional liability insurance coverage for individual claims up to $1 million (subject to a deductible of $100,000 per claim). Riverview is self-insured for amounts above $1 million but less than $5 million. Any liability award in excess of $5 million is covered by a commercial liability policy; for example, the policy pays $2 million on a $7 million award. The hospital is currently involved in eight suits involving claims of various amounts that could ultimately be tried before juries. Although it is impossible to determine the exact potential liability in these claims, management does not believe that the settlement of these cases would have a material effect on the hospital's financial position.

Assume that you have just joined the staff of Riverview Community Hospital as a special assistant to the CEO. On your first day on the job, the CEO, Melissa Randolph, stated that the best way to get to know the financial and operating condition of the hospital is to conduct a thorough financial statement and operating indicator analysis; thus, she assigned you the task. Although you also believe that this is a good way to get started, you wonder whether Melissa has any ulterior motives. Perhaps the hospital is having problems and she thinks that you can spot them or perhaps she wants to test your analytical skills. Melissa is from the "old school" of hospital management and has been looking for someone to bring modern management methods to the hospital.

In any event, she has already scheduled a financial and operating performance analysis presentation at the next board of trustees meeting as a way for you to meet the board members. To help you structure your presentation, Melissa suggested that you make the following points:

1. Interpret the hospital's statements of cash flows.
2. Present an overview of the hospital's financial position using the Du Pont equation as a guide.
3. Use ratio analysis to identify the hospital's specific financial strengths and weaknesses. But, she warned, the board is not going to appreciate a lengthy dialogue with too many individual ratios. Focus on key findings and one or two ratios per category—don't put them to sleep! Also, use graphs or other techniques to summarize the data.
4. Use operating indicator analysis to identify the operational factors that explain the hospital's current financial condition.
5. Summarize your evaluation of the hospital's financial condition. However, **don't just rehash the numbers**; rather, present your views on the potential underlying economic and managerial factors that might have caused any problems that surfaced in the financial and operating analysis.
6. Make any recommendations that you believe the hospital should follow to ensure future financial soundness.

In preparing for the presentation, several relevant factors came to light. First, in reviewing the policy decisions made by Riverview's board of trustees over the past decade, you found out that in 2004 the board made the decision to significantly expand the hospital's outpatient services. The rationale was that many procedures that historically were done on an inpatient basis were now being done in an outpatient setting, and if Riverview did not offer such services it would lose the patients to other providers.

Second, you discovered that board members were complaining that too much time is being spent at quarterly board meetings discussing the hospital's financial condition. "There is so much to accomplish," said one member, "that we just don't have the time to consider a large number of ratios at each meeting."

You know that many healthcare providers are now using dashboards to focus on key performance indicators (KPIs). A dashboard is nothing more than a way to summarize an organization's financial and operating performance. Of course, the name stems from an automobile's dashboard, which contains gauges that give drivers essential information about the car's performance and operating condition. Thus, you plan to develop two dashboards, each containing **no more than five KPIs**. One dashboard will use financial ratios to focus on financial performance, while the other will use operating indicator ratios to focus on operating performance. You plan to present your recommendations for the contents of these dashboards, along with the rationale for the ratios chosen, at the board meeting. Your ultimate goal is to replace the full financial and operating performance discussion at future board meetings with a limited discussion of the KPIs.

The day before your presentation, Melissa stopped you in the hallway. In addition to asking if you are ready to go, she asked whether or not the board should be concerned about the hospital's annual economic value added (EVA) performance. Apparently, she just read an article in *Fortune* magazine that discusses this measure of managerial performance. (For more information on EVA, as well as market value added [MVA], see the Stern Stewart & Co. website at www.eva.com.) Then she said, "By the way, our overall (corporate) cost of capital is 10 percent." You are not quite sure why she passed that information on to you, but you jotted it down just in case.

EXHIBIT 1.1
Riverview Community Hospital: Statements of Operations (millions of dollars)

	2005	2006	2007	2008	2009
Revenues					
Net patient service revenue	$25.661	$27.236	$28.796	$30.576	$34.582
Other revenue	1.305	1.261	1.237	1.853	1.834
Total revenues	$26.966	$28.497	$30.033	$32.429	$36.416
Expenses					
Salaries and wages	$10.829	$11.135	$12.245	$12.468	$13.994
Fringe benefits	1.496	1.731	1.830	2.408	2.568
Interest expense	1.341	1.305	1.181	1.598	1.776
Depreciation	1.708	1.977	2.350	2.658	2.778
Provision for bad debts	0.546	0.589	0.622	0.655	0.776
Professional liability	0.102	0.157	0.140	0.201	0.218
Other	7.874	8.389	9.036	10.339	11.848
Total expenses	$23.896	$25.283	$27.404	$30.327	$33.958
Excess of revenues over expenses	$ 3.070	$ 3.214	$ 2.629	$ 2.102	$ 2.458

EXHIBIT 1.2
Riverview Community Hospital: Balance Sheets (millions of dollars)

	2005	2006	2007	2008	2009
Assets					
Cash and investments	$ 3.513	$ 5.799	$ 4.673	$ 5.069	$ 2.795
Accounts receivable (net)	5.915	4.832	4.359	5.674	7.413
Inventories	0.338	0.403	0.432	0.523	0.601
Other current assets	0.693	0.294	0.308	0.703	0.923
Total current assets	$10.459	$11.328	$ 9.772	$11.969	$11.732
Gross plant and equipment	$37.999	$42.005	$47.786	$55.333	$59.552
Accumulated depreciation	8.831	10.092	11.820	14.338	17.009
Net plant and equipment	$29.168	$31.913	$35.966	$40.995	$42.543
Total assets	$39.627	$43.241	$45.738	$52.964	$54.275
Liabilities and Net Assets					
Accounts payable	$ 1.068	$ 1.273	$ 0.928	$ 1.253	$ 1.760
Accruals	0.692	0.942	1.460	1.503	1.176
Current portion of LT debt	0.136	0.290	0.110	1.341	1.465
Total current liabilities	$ 1.896	$ 2.505	$ 2.498	$ 4.097	$ 4.401
Long-term debt	15.959	15.775	15.673	19.222	17.795
Net assets	21.772	24.961	27.567	29.645	32.079
Total liabilities and net assets	$39.627	$43.241	$45.738	$52.964	$54.275

EXHIBIT 1.3
Riverview Community Hospital: Statements of Cash Flows (millions of dollars)

	2006	2007	2008	2009
Cash Flows from Operating Activities				
Income from operations	$3.214	$2.629	$2.102	$2.458
Noncash expenses	1.952	2.326	2.633	2.756
Change in accounts receivable	1.083	0.473	(1.315)	(1.739)
Change in inventories	(0.065)	(0.029)	(0.091)	(0.078)
Change in other current assets	0.399	(0.014)	(0.395)	(0.220)
Change in accounts payable	0.205	(0.345)	0.325	0.507
Change in accruals	0.250	0.518	0.043	(0.327)
Change in current portion of LT debt	0.154	(0.180)	1.231	0.124
Net cash flow from operations	$7.192	$5.378	$4.533	$3.481
Cash Flows from Investing Activities				
Fixed asset acquisitions	($4.722)	($6.402)	($7.686)	($4.328)
Cash Flows from Financing Activities				
Increase (decrease) in LT debt	($0.184)	($0.102)	$3.549	($1.427)
Net increase (decrease) in cash	$2.286	($1.126)	$0.396	($2.274)
Beginning cash and investments	$3.513	$5.799	$4.673	$5.069
Ending cash and investments	$5.799	$4.673	$5.069	$2.795

LT: long term
Note: The noncash expenses and fixed asset acquisitions data in the statements of cash flows are somewhat different than they would be if calculated directly from the other financial statements because of asset revaluations.

EXHIBIT 1.4
Riverview Community Hospital: Selected Operating Data

	2005	2006	2007	2008	2009
Medicare discharges	3,008	2,960	2,721	2,860	2,741
Total discharges	9,680	9,311	8,784	8,318	8,576
Outpatient visits	30,754	31,960	32,285	32,878	36,796
Licensed beds	210	210	210	210	210
Staffed beds	192	196	193	197	178
Patient days	45,296	45,983	44,085	42,434	40,062
Case mix index	1.2531	1.2674	1.2869	1.2993	1.3161
Full-time equivalents	604.5	618.1	610.8	625.8	619.3

EXHIBIT 1.5
2009 Selected Industry Financial Data (200–299 Beds)

	+Quartile	Median	−Quartile
Profitability Ratios			
Deductible ratio*	0.34	0.26	0.18
Profit (total) margin	5.58%	3.48%	0.53%
Return on assets	5.80%	3.10%	0.40%
Return on equity	15.66%	6.01%	0.62%
Liquidity Ratios			
Current ratio	2.53	1.99	1.48
Days cash on hand	32.35	15.89	6.24
Debt Management Ratios			
Debt ratio	62.90%	48.40%	35.20%
LT debt to equity	127.00%	64.70%	26.90%
Times interest earned	4.29	2.23	1.14
Fixed charge coverage	2.18	1.35	1.02
Cash flow coverage	5.32	3.22	1.76
Asset Management Ratios			
Inventory turnover	98.68	63.95	43.99
Current asset turnover	3.94	3.38	2.88
Fixed asset turnover	2.20	1.76	1.49
Total asset turnover	1.04	0.89	0.75
Average collection period (days)	87.53	75.67	63.33
Average payment period (days)	71.24	56.52	45.84
Other Ratios			
Average age of plant (years)	8.86	7.39	6.14

*Deductions/Gross patient service revenue
LT: long term
Notes: 1. The industry data shown here are for illustrative purposes only and hence should not be used outside this case.

2. The upper quartile is based on the higher numerical value for the ratio and the lower quartile on the lower numerical value, regardless of whether a high value is good or bad. The interpretation is left to the analyst.

EXHIBIT 1.6
2009 Selected Industry Operating Data (200–299 Beds)

	+Quartile	Median	−Quartile
Profit Indicators			
Profit per discharge[a]	$89.04	($21.30)	($120.08)
Profit per visit[b]	$ 6.22	$ 0.66	($ 7.01)
Net Price Indicators			
Net price per discharge	$4,091	$3,411	$ 2,815
Net price per visit	$ 201	$ 139	$ 98
Medicare payment percentage	43.47%	36.60%	31.25%
Bad debt/charity percentage[c]	7.89%	4.76%	2.97%
Contractual allowance %[d]	25.27%	20.02%	12.12%
Outpatient revenue %	25.26%	21.03%	17.44%
Volume Indicators			
Occupancy rate	67.12%	58.10%	47.84%
Average daily census[e]	173.23	144.73	114.39
Length of Stay Indicators			
Average length of stay (days)	6.80	6.07	5.41
Adjusted length of stay[f]	6.48	5.36	4.52
Intensity of Service Indicators			
Cost per discharge	$ 3,937	$ 3,392	$ 2,972
Adjusted cost per discharge[g]	$ 3,417	$ 2,924	$ 2,572
Cost per visit[h]	$202.23	$141.97	$111.53
Case mix index	1.2795	1.1756	1.0259
Efficiency Indicators			
FTEs per occupied bed	4.59	4.15	3.77
Outpatient man-hours per visit[i]	4.68	5.84	8.66
Unit Cost Indicators			
Salary per FTE[j]	$24,447	$22,517	$20,347
Employee benefits percentage[k]	19.58%	17.04%	15.18%
Liability costs per discharge[l]	$ 80.94	$ 42.05	$ 18.31

[a](Net inpatient revenue − Inpatient cost)/Total discharges
[b](Net outpatient revenue − Outpatient cost)/Total visits

**EXHIBIT 1.6
(continued)
Selected Industry
Operating Data**

c(Bad debt + Charity care)/Gross patient revenue
dContractual allowances/Gross patient revenue
ePatient days/365
fAverage length of stay/Case mix index
gCost per discharge/Case mix index
hTotal outpatient expenses/Total outpatient visits
i(Outpatient FTEs x 2,080)/Total visits
jTotal salaries/FTEs
kFringe benefit costs/Total salaries
lInpatient professional liability costs/Total discharges

FTE: full-time equivalent

Notes: 1. The industry data shown here are for illustrative purposes only and hence should not be used outside this case.

2. The upper quartile is based on the higher numerical value for the ratio and the lower quartile on the lower numerical value, regardless of whether a high value is good or bad. The interpretation is left to the analyst.

CHESAPEAKE HEALTH PLANS
ASSESSING HMO PERFORMANCE

2

CHESAPEAKE HEALTH PLANS is one of Virginia's largest managed care organizations (MCOs). In fact, it is the largest of the state's not-for-profit MCOs. It offers prepaid health coverage to more than 400,000 members in 15 counties, including the following major cities: Richmond, Norfolk, Virginia Beach, Arlington, Alexandria, and Roanoke.

Chesapeake's various products include commercial health maintenance organizations (HMOs), preferred provider organizations (PPOs), and point of service (POS) plans as well as Medicare HMOs (Medicare Advantage Plans), which are all designed to meet the needs of a wide segment of Virginia's population of approximately 8 million. The breakdown of plan types is as follows:

Plan Type	Percent of Revenue
Commercial HMO	46
Medicare HMO	39
PPO	10
POS	5
	100

Chesapeake was the first HMO in Virginia to seek and receive accreditation from the National Committee for Quality Assurance (NCQA), and each of its component plans has the highest accreditation level: excellent. NCQA judges HMOs on how well they comply with more than 60 standards and performance measures that fall into broad categories such as access and service, provider qualifications, and staying healthy. Some of the evaluation focuses on systems and processes, but accreditation results also depend on clinical performance as measured by HEDIS (Health Plan Employer Data and Information Set) and patient satisfaction as measured by CAHPS (Consumer Assessment of Healthcare Providers and Systems). (For more information on the NCQA, visit its website at www.ncqa.org.)

A summary of Chesapeake's 2008 and 2009 HMO plan financial data is presented in Exhibit 2.1, while Exhibit 2.2 contains a summary of operating and enrollment data. To help in analyzing Chesapeake's performance, its managers have classified the following four Virginia HMOs as "primary competitors."

HMO	Number of Counties Served	2009 Total Enrollment	2009 Total Assets (000s)
WellLife	23	516,858	$408,707
Signet Healthcare	15	360,252	178,662
Proxima	15	247,109	144,982
Sparta	28	205,296	103,504

These plans have the geographic coverage and financial resources to be prominent players in the Virginia managed care industry. Furthermore, the primary competitors are operating in the same service areas and have a similar product mix as Chesapeake and hence are potential threats to its future success. In addition to comparisons to national data, all internal analyses that use benchmarking compare Chesapeake's performance to the state average as well as to the primary competitor list. **Note, however, that not all relevant performance measures have a complete set of comparative data available.**

Exhibit 2.3 contains selected financial and operating ratios for Chesapeake's primary competitors as well as the means and medians for all Virginia HMOs. Exhibit 2.4 contains selected national data. Note that all comparative data are for HMO plans only. Data relevant to competitors' other plans, such as PPO and POS plans, are not available. Exhibit 2.5 contains selected ratio definitions. (For a better understanding of the types of comparative data available for managed care plans, see the Health Leaders-InterStudy website at www.hmo-data.com.)

Assume that you have just started an administrative residency at Chesapeake Health Plans. On your first day at the organization, Charles Redman, the chief executive officer, stated that the best way to get to know the financial and operating condition of any business is to do a brief financial statement and operating indicator analysis; thus, he assigned you the task. Although you agree that this is a great way to learn more about Chesapeake and its competitors, you wonder whether he has any hidden motives. Perhaps the company is having financial problems and he thinks that you can spot them, or perhaps he just wants to test your analytical skills.

In any event, he has already scheduled a financial and operating performance analysis presentation for the next executive committee meeting as a way for you to demonstrate your skills to Chesapeake's senior managers. In preparing for the meeting, you called Jennifer Wall, the previous administrative resident, to get some hints on how to prepare for your presentation to the executive committee. Jennifer just left Chesapeake for a great job with Humana. Her advice was to do a standard financial statement analysis, including statement of cash flows analysis, Du Pont analysis, and ratio and operating indicator analyses.

As you began the analysis, it became apparent that the ratios used and their interpretations differ across industries; that is, the ratios that are critical to identifying the financial condition of a hospital are not necessarily the same as the ratios that are critical to a managed care plan. In addition, many of the ratios that are relevant to both hospitals and managed care plans have values that differ substantially. To help the executive committee in interpreting your presentation, you plan to point out key differences between your analysis for a health plan and that for a hospital as they occur. Last, you know that identifying key areas of concern and recommending courses of action are more important than merely going over the numbers.

EXHIBIT 2.1
Chesapeake Health Plans:
HMO Plan Financial Data
(millions of dollars)

	2008	2009
Statements of Operations		
Premium revenue	$313.7	$357.6
Interest income	2.4	3.5
Total revenues	$316.1	$361.1
Operating expenses:		
Medical costs	$263.0	$291.8
Selling and administrative	36.8	43.6
Depreciation	4.7	5.0
Total operating expenses	$304.5	$340.4
Net income	$ 11.6	$ 20.7
Balance Sheets		
Cash	$ 37.2	$ 27.2
Marketable securities	42.7	60.9
Premiums receivable	3.7	7.4
Total current assets	$ 83.6	$ 95.5
Net fixed assets	30.0	31.7
Total assets	$113.6	$127.2
Medical costs payable	$ 44.8	$ 48.7
Accounts payable/accruals	15.4	17.3
Total current liabilities	$ 60.2	$ 66.0
Long-term debt	17.1	4.2
Net assets (equity)	36.3	57.0
Total liabilities and net assets	$113.6	$127.2
Other Data		
Medical loss ratio	83.8%	81.6%
Administrative cost ratio	13.2%	13.6%
Total commercial premium revenue	$170.9	$205.6
Total Medicare revenue	$142.8	$152.0
Total physician services expense	$125.6	$127.1
Total inpatient expense	$ 80.8	$ 90.1
Total other medical expense	$ 56.6	$ 74.6

	2008	2009
Commercial premium revenue PMPM	$127.82	$127.90
Medicare revenue PMPM	$449.37	$437.23
Commercial patient days per 1,000 enrollees	302.9	266.4
Medicare patient days per 1,000 enrollees	1,622.4	1,418.1
Commercial member–months	1,337,036	1,607,036
Commercial physician encounters	594,381	622,749
Commercial inpatient days	43,661	39,763
Medicare member–months	317,778	347,643
Medicare physician encounters	149,622	185,283

PMPM: per member per month

EXHIBIT 2.2 Chesapeake Health Plans: HMO Plan Operating and Enrollment Data

	2008	2009
Total Margin		
WellLife	4.8%	5.8%
Signet Healthcare	3.0	3.2
Proxima	9.1	(0.7)
Sparta	10.5	9.1
State average	3.8	(3.9)
State median	4.8	4.7
Percent Administrative Expense		
WellLife	12.1%	11.5%
Signet Healthcare	12.2	13.4
Proxima	13.6	16.4
Sparta	23.9	26.8
State average	15.5	17.4
State median	14.8	15.7
Percent Inpatient Expense		
WellLife	32.2%	30.3%
Signet Healthcare	22.8	22.4
Proxima	21.2	23.0
Sparta	18.2	18.8
State average	25.2	23.3
State median	23.6	24.3

EXHIBIT 2.3 Selected State HMO Industry Financial and Operating Data (millions of dollars)

EXHIBIT 2.3 (continued)
Selected State HMO Industry Financial and Operating Data (millions of dollars)

	2008	2009
Percent Physician Expense		
WellLife	54.1%	56.9%
Signet Healthcare	31.3	30.3
Proxima	22.7	24.9
Sparta	12.8	18.6
State average	28.8	31.3
State median	31.1	31.6
Percent Other Medical Expense		
WellLife	0.1%	0.1%
Signet Healthcare	8.9	7.8
Proxima	27.5	30.2
Sparta	45.7	35.0
State average	14.6	12.5
State median	10.2	8.9
Commercial Premium Revenue PMPM		
WellLife	$108.68	$110.19
Signet Healthcare	39.86	27.50
Proxima	120.68	124.27
Sparta	88.41	95.06
State average	101.17	102.53
State median	108.32	108.95
Medicare Revenue PMPM		
WellLife	$406.57	$421.57
Signet Healthcare	N/A	N/A
Proxima	N/A	N/A
Sparta	N/A	N/A
State average	365.12	376.04
State median	426.18	430.57
Commercial Inpatient Days per 1,000 Enrollees		
WellLife	245.4	246.0
Signet Healthcare	258.4	248.8
Proxima	251.8	259.2
Sparta	198.2	248.9
State average	278.0	237.0
State median	279.1	248.8

EXHIBIT 2.3 (continued) Selected State HMO Industry Financial and Operating Data (millions of dollars)

	2008	2009
Medicare Inpatient Days per 1,000 Enrollees		
WellLife	1,388.4	1,323.8
Signet Healthcare	1,165.2	1,188.7
Proxima	1,518.8	1,382.2
Sparta	1,623.8	1,566.9
State average	1,432.1	1,375.5
State median	1,380.5	1,350.6
Commercial Physician Encounters per Member		
WellLife	2.2	3.6
Signet Healthcare	1.5	1.4
Proxima	2.7	2.6
Sparta	3.5	3.6
State average	3.8	3.8
State median	3.9	3.7
Medicare Physician Encounters per Member		
WellLife	9.8	9.6
Signet Healthcare	6.6	6.9
Proxima	10.1	10.0
Sparta	11.2	11.3
State average	9.1	9.1
State median	8.6	8.9

Note: The Virginia data for the HMO industry contained in this table are for illustrative purposes only. These data should not be used to conduct actual financial analyses.

EXHIBIT 2.4
Selected 2009 National HMO Industry Financial and Operating Data

Average copay per office visit	$ 8
Average copay per hospitalization	$36
Average copay per pharmacy prescription	$ 7
Medical loss ratio	
Upper quartile	89.0%
Median	84.9
Lower quartile	80.0
Administrative cost ratio	
Upper quartile	14.4%
Median	12.0
Lower quartile	9.0
Operating margin	
Upper quartile	5.0%
Median	2.5
Lower quartile	1.1
Total margin	
Upper quartile	5.5%
Median	2.9
Lower quartile	1.5
Return on assets (ROA)	
Upper quartile	16.5%
Median	11.3
Lower quartile	4.8
Return on equity (ROE)	
Upper quartile	50.2%
Median	31.4
Lower quartile	18.2
Current ratio	
Upper quartile	1.29
Median	0.95
Lower quartile	0.49
Days cash on hand	
Upper quartile	32.7
Median	10.3
Lower quartile	0.8

EXHIBIT 2.4 (continued) Selected 2009 National HMO Industry Financial and Operating Data

Current asset turnover
- Upper quartile   14.1
- Median   6.4
- Lower quartile   3.7

Total asset turnover
- Upper quartile   4.1
- Median   3.1
- Lower quartile   2.2

Days premiums receivable
- Upper quartile   14.0
- Median   8.9
- Lower quartile   7.0

Debt ratio
- Upper quartile   81.3%
- Median   68.4
- Lower quartile   59.7

Note: The national data for the HMO industry contained in this table are for illustrative purposes only. These data should not be used to conduct actual financial analyses.

**EXHIBIT 2.5
Selected Ratio
Definitions**

Medical Loss Ratio

$$\frac{\text{Medical expenses}}{\text{Premium revenue}}$$

Administrative Cost Ratio

$$\frac{\text{Selling and administrative expenses + Depreciation}}{\text{Premium revenue}}$$

Operating Margin

$$\frac{\text{Net income − Interest income}}{\text{Premium revenue}}$$

Percent Administrative Expense

$$\frac{\text{Selling and administrative expense}}{\text{Total operating expenses}}$$

Percent Inpatient Expense

$$\frac{\text{Inpatient expense}}{\text{Total operating expenses}}$$

Percent Physician Expense

$$\frac{\text{Physician services expense}}{\text{Total operating expenses}}$$

Percent Other Medical Expense

$$\frac{\text{Other medical expense}}{\text{Total operating expenses}}$$

*Managerial
Accounting*

RIO GRANDE MEDICAL CENTER

COST ALLOCATION CONCEPTS

RIO GRANDE MEDICAL CENTER is a full-service not-for-profit acute care hospital with 325 beds located in Rio Grande, Texas. The bulk of the hospital's facilities are devoted to inpatient care and emergency services. However, a 100,000-square-foot section of the hospital complex is devoted to outpatient services. Currently, this space has two primary uses. About 80 percent of the space is used by the Outpatient Clinic, which handles all routine outpatient services offered by the hospital. The remaining 20 percent is used by the Dialysis Center.

The Dialysis Center performs hemodialysis and peritoneal dialysis, which are alternative processes that remove wastes and excess water from the blood for patients with end-stage renal (kidney) disease. In hemodialysis, blood is pumped from the patient's arm through a shunt into a dialysis machine, which uses a cleansing solution and an artificial membrane to perform the functions of a healthy kidney. Then, the cleansed blood is pumped back into the patient through a second shunt.

In peritoneal dialysis, the cleansing solution is inserted directly into the abdominal cavity through a catheter. The body naturally cleanses the blood through the peritoneum—a thin membrane that lines the abdominal cavity.

Typically, hemodialysis patients require three dialyses a week, with each treatment lasting about four hours. Patients who use peritoneal dialysis change their own cleansing solutions at home, usually about six times per day. This procedure can be done manually when active or automatically by machine when sleeping. However, the patient's overall condition, as well as the positioning of the catheter, must be monitored regularly at the Dialysis Center.

Rio Grande's new cost accounting system, which was installed two years ago, allocates facilities costs (which at Rio Grande essentially consist of building depreciation and interest on long-term debt) on the basis of square footage. Currently, the facilities cost allocation rate is $15 per square foot, so the facilities cost allocation is 20,000 x $15 = $300,000 for the Dialysis Center and 80,000 x $15 = $1,200,000 for the Outpatient Clinic. All other overhead costs, such as administration, finance, maintenance, and housekeeping, are lumped together and called "general overhead." These costs are allocated on the basis of 10 percent of the revenues of each patient service department. The current allocation of general overhead is $270,000 for the Dialysis Center and $1,600,000 for the Outpatient Clinic, which results in total overhead allocations of $570,000 for the Dialysis Center and $2,800,000 for the Outpatient Clinic.

Recent growth in volume of the Outpatient Clinic has created a need for 25 percent more space than is currently assigned. Because the Outpatient Clinic is much larger than the Dialysis Center, and because its patients need frequent access to other departments within the hospital, the decision was made to keep the Outpatient Clinic in its current location and to move the Dialysis Center to another location to free up space within the hospital complex. Such a move would give the Outpatient Clinic 100,000 square feet, a 25 percent increase.

After attempting to find space for the Dialysis Center within the hospital complex, it was soon determined that a new 20,000-square-foot building must be built. This building would be situated three blocks away from the hospital complex, in a location that would be much more convenient for dialysis patients (and Center employees) because of ease of parking. The 20,000 square feet of space, which can be more efficiently used than the old space, allows for some increase in patient volume, although it is unclear whether or not the move will generate additional dialysis patients.

Construction cost of the new building is estimated at $120 per square foot, for a total cost of $2,400,000. Additionally, land, furniture, and other fittings, along with relocation of equipment, files, and other items, would cost $1,600,000, for a total cost of $4,000,000. The $4,000,000 cost would be financed by a 7.75 percent, 20-year first-mortgage loan. When both the principal amount (which can be considered depreciation) and interest are amortized over 20 years, the end result is an annual cost of financing of $400,000. Thus, it is possible to estimate the actual annual facilities costs for the new Dialysis Center, something that is not possible for units located within the hospital complex.

Exhibit 3.1 contains the projected profit and loss (P&L) statement for the Dialysis Center before adjusting for the move. Rio Grande's department heads receive annual bonuses on the basis of each department's contribution to the hospital's bottom line (profit). In the past, only direct costs were considered, but Rio Grande's CEO has decided that bonuses would now be based on full (total) costs.

The new approach to awarding bonuses, coupled with the potential for increases in indirect cost allocation, is of great concern to John Van Pelt, the director of the Dialysis Center. Under the current allocation of indirect costs (see Exhibit 3.1), John would have a reasonable chance at an end-of-year bonus, as the forecast puts the Dialysis Center in the black. However, any increase in the indirect cost allocation would likely put him out of the money.

At the next department heads' meeting, John voiced his concern about the impact of any allocation changes on the Dialysis Center's profitability, so Rio Grande's CEO asked the chief financial officer (CFO), Rick Simmons, to look into the matter. In essence, the CEO said that the final allocation is up to Rick but that any allocation changes must be made within outpatient services. In other words, any change in indirect cost allocation to the Dialysis Center must be offset by an equal, but opposite, change in the allocation to the Outpatient Clinic.

To get started, Rick created Exhibit 3.2. In creating the exhibit, Rick assumed that the new Dialysis Center would have the same number of stations as the old one, would serve the same number of patients, and would receive the same reimbursement rates. Also, direct operating expenses would differ only slightly from the current situation because the same personnel and equipment would be used. Thus, for all practical purposes, the revenues and direct costs of the Dialysis Center would be unaffected by the move.

The data in Exhibit 3.2 for the expanded Outpatient Clinic are based on the assumption that the expansion would allow volume to increase by 25 percent and that both revenues and direct costs would increase by a like amount. Furthermore, to keep the analysis manageable, the assumption was made that the overall hospital allocation rates for both facilities costs and general overhead would not materially change because of the expansion.

Rick knew that his "trial balloon" allocation, which is shown in Exhibit 3.2 in the columns labeled "Initial Allocation," would create some controversy. In the past, facilities costs were aggregated, so all departments were charged a cost based on the average embedded (historical) cost regardless of the actual age (or value) of the space occupied. Thus, a basement room with no windows was allocated the same facilities costs (per square foot) as was the fifth floor executive suite. Because many department heads thought this approach was unfair, Rick wanted to begin allocating facilities overhead on a true cost basis. Thus, in his initial allocation, Rick used actual facilities costs as the basis for the allocation to the Dialysis Center.

Needless to say, John's response to the initial allocation was less than enthusiastic. Specifically, he raised these points:

1. Is it fair for the Dialysis Center to suffer (in profitability) from the move even though it had nothing to do with it?
2. Should the Dialysis Center be charged actual facilities costs for its new location? After all, the move was forced by the Outpatient Clinic, which is being charged for facilities at the lower average allocation rate. Under the concept of charging for actual facilities costs, department heads might be better off resisting proposed moves to new (and potentially more efficient) facilities because such moves would result in increased facilities allocations.
3. Even if the true cost concept were applied to the Dialysis Center, is the $400,000 annual allocation amount correct? After all, the building has a useful life that is probably significantly longer than 20 years—the life of the loan used to determine the allocation amount. If the true cost concept is applied, what would be the allocation in the 21st year, after the mortgage had been paid off?

4. The revenue that the Dialysis Center "receives" from patient use of the pharmacy appears to be passed on directly to the pharmacy. That is, the Dialysis Center books $800,000 in annual revenue but then is charged $800,000 for the drugs used. Should this "revenue" be counted when general overhead allocations are made? To make his point, John discovered that the pharmacy supplies used for dialysis actually cost the pharmacy $400,000, so the pharmacy makes a profit of $400,000 on drugs that are actually "sold" by the Dialysis Center.

Before Rick was able to respond to John's concerns, he suddenly left Rio Grande to be the CFO of a competing investor-owned hospital. The task of completing the allocation study was given to you, Rio Grande's current administrative resident. You remember that to be of most benefit to the organization, cost allocations should (1) be perceived as being fair by the parties involved and (2) promote overall cost savings within the organization. However, you also realize that in practice cost allocation is complex and somewhat arbitrary. Some department heads argue that the best approach to overhead allocations is the "Marxist approach," by which allocations are based on each patient service department's ability to cover overhead costs.

Considering all the relevant issues, you must develop and justify a new indirect cost allocation scheme for outpatient services. Summarize your results in the "Alternative Allocation" columns in Exhibit 3.2, and be prepared to justify your recommendations at the next department heads' meeting.

EXHIBIT 3.1
Rio Grande Medical Center Dialysis Center: Pro Forma P&L Statement Assuming Status Quo

Revenues	
Hemodialysis program	$ 1,300,000
Peritoneal dialysis program	600,000
Pharmaceutical supplies	800,000
Total revenues	$ 2,700,000
Direct Expenses	
Salaries and benefits	$ 900,000
Pharmaceutical supplies	800,000
Other medical/administrative supplies	100,000
Utilities	80,000
Lease expense	120,000
Other expenses	100,000
Total expenses	$ 2,100,000
Net gain (loss) before indirect costs	$ 600,000
Indirect Expenses	
Facilities costs	$ 300,000
General overhead	270,000
Total overhead costs	$ 570,000
Net profit	$ 30,000

Note: Pharmacy revenues are based on reimbursement amounts, not costs.

EXHIBIT 3.2
Rio Grande Medical Center: Dialysis Center (DC) and Outpatient Clinic (OC) Summary Projections

P&L Statements:	Without Expansion		With Expansion			
			Initial Allocation		Alternative Allocation	
	DC	OC	DC	OC	DC	OC
Revenues/Direct Costs						
Total revenues	$ 2,700,000	$16,000,000	$ 2,700,000	$20,000,000	$ 2,700,000	$20,000,000
Direct expenses	2,100,000	9,833,155	2,100,000	12,291,444	2,100,000	12,291,444
Contribution margin	$ 600,000	$ 6,166,845	$ 600,000	$ 7,708,556	$ 600,000	$ 7,708,556
Percent of revenues	22.2%	38.5%	22.2%	38.5%	22.2%	38.5%
Indirect Costs						
Facilities costs	$ 300,000	$ 1,200,000	$ 400,000	$ 1,500,000	$	$
General overhead	270,000	1,600,000	270,000	2,000,000		
Total overhead	$ 570,000	$ 2,800,000	$ 670,000	$ 3,500,000	$	$
Net profit	$ 30,000	$ 3,366,845	($ 70,000)	$ 4,208,556	$	$
Percent of revenues	1.1%	21.0%	(2.6%)	21.0%	%	%
Facilities Cost Allocation:						
Square footage	20,000	80,000	20,000	100,000	20,000	100,000
Facilities costs per square foot	$ 15.00	$ 15.00	$ 20.00	$ 15.00	$	$
Other Overhead Allocation:						
General overhead costs as a % of revenue	10.0%	10.0%	10.0%	10.0%	%	%

Note: The term "contribution margin" as used here means the amount available to cover overhead costs, as opposed to the traditional meaning of the amount available to cover fixed costs.

APPLE VALLEY FAMILY PRACTICE

COST ALLOCATION METHODS

4

Apple Valley Family Practice (the Group) is a medical practice with four locations in the Minneapolis/St. Paul area. The clinical staff consists of 20 physicians, all of whom practice in one or more areas of family medicine, and 46 physician extenders and nurses. The Group is organized into three patient services departments: Adult Medicine, Obstetrics, and Pediatrics. Supporting these patient service departments are three support departments: Administration, Facilities, and Finance. Exhibit 4.1 contains the Group's summary revenue and cost projections by department for the coming year.

As part of a much-needed overhaul of the cost allocation process, the Group contracted with a major accounting firm to estimate the amount of services provided by the support departments to each other and to each patient service department. The intent of the study was to provide data that would help the Group develop a better cost allocation system than could the outdated, arbitrary system currently in use. The results of this study are contained in Exhibit 4.2. Although expressed as percentages of the total dollar amount of support provided to other departments (instead of the more typical cost allocation rates), the data in Exhibit 4.2 are based on an extensive study using sound managerial accounting techniques. Thus, both senior management and department heads at the Group are comfortable with the resulting allocation percentages. (Hint: To ensure that you apply the percentages properly, pay attention to Note 2 at the bottom of Exhibit 4.2.)

The second step in the cost allocation process improvement initiative is to choose the allocation method. Four allocation methods are under consideration: direct, step-down, double apportionment, and reciprocal. To aid in the decision, George Poulis, the Group's CFO, has asked Mary Jansen, the Group's administrative resident, to conduct a study and to make a recommendation regarding the best allocation method.

This task can be approached several ways, but Mary has decided to "examine by doing." That is, she plans to use the data in Exhibits 4.1 and 4.2 to determine the overhead cost allocations under each method. Once this is done, she will be able to compare and contrast the results.

Of course, the final decision cannot be made without considering the costs involved in implementing each allocation method. When Mary asked George about the costs inherent in each allocation method, George said, "I don't know! Assume that the direct method is the least costly, the reciprocal method is the most costly, and the other two fall somewhere in between." He also expects Mary to make some judgments on the relative profitability of the patient services departments under the recommended allocation system.

Mary began her analysis by reviewing the allocation methods presented in her old healthcare finance textbook. She had no problem remembering basic cost allocation concepts, but she did hit two snags.

The first problem was that the textbook did not describe the double apportionment method. However, after a little research, Mary discovered that the double apportionment method is a slightly more complicated version of the step-down method. In essence, the double apportionment method first recognizes support provided by service departments to all other service departments as well as to the patient services departments. After this step, which is called the first allocation (apportionment), some costs still remain in the support departments. Then, a second apportionment, which uses the step-down method, is used to move all remaining support department costs to the patient services departments. In this method, service department support to all other service departments is recognized. In the pure step-down method, on the other hand, service department support is recognized only to "downstream" service departments.

Here's how Mary assumed that the double apportionment method would be applied to the Group: (This allocation method can be applied in other ways.)

- First, direct Administration costs would be allocated to the other five departments (two support and three patient services).
- Second, direct Facilities costs would be allocated to all other departments (including Administration and Finance).
- Third, direct Finance costs would be allocated to all other departments (including Administration and Facilities).

After these three allocations are completed, the first apportionment is finished. Some costs still remain in the support departments—the intra-support department allocations from the first apportionment—so a second apportionment is necessary. The second apportionment is conducted using the step-down method as it is normally applied, except that the application of the first apportionment means that the starting cost pool values are much lower.

The second problem was that Mary did not know how to perform the reciprocal allocation. One method is to use simultaneous equations (but higher mathematics has never been Mary's strong suit), while the second method uses an iterative approach. Fortunately, Mary had recently read an article in *Accounting Monthly* that included an Excel model that uses the iterative approach to accomplish reciprocal allocation. To help with the analysis, Mary created a new spreadsheet model, which uses the Group's numbers, to calculate the allocation not only for the reciprocal method but also for the other three methods.

Assume that you are in Mary's shoes. Complete her assignment and prepare a report to present to the Group's executive committee. In addition to merely completing the task as it stands, you decide to assess the sensitivity of the results to (1) the relative sizes of the direct costs at each support department and (2) the amount of support provided by the support departments to each other. Exhibit 4.3 contains the values that you intend to use in your sensitivity analysis.

**EXHIBIT 4.1
Apple Valley
Family Practice:
Departmental Revenue
and Cost Projections**

Revenues	
Adult Medicine	$12,000,000
Obstetrics	6,000,000
Pediatrics	2,000,000
Total revenues	$20,000,000
Direct Costs	
Patient Services	
Adult Medicine	$ 6,000,000
Obstetrics	3,600,000
Pediatrics	1,200,000
Subtotal	$10,800,000
Support	
Administration	1,000,000
Facilities	4,400,000
Finance	1,800,000
Subtotal	$ 7,200,000
Total expenses	$18,000,000
Pre-tax profit	$ 2,000,000

EXHIBIT 4.2
Apple Valley Family Practice:
Allocation Percentages

	Percentage of Services Provided by		
Services Provided to	Administration	Facilities	Finance
Administration	—	5%	5%
Facilities	10%	—	5
Finance	10	10	—
Adult Medicine	35	55	50
Obstetrics	20	10	25
Pediatrics	25	20	15
Total	100%	100%	100%
Percentage to support departments	20%	15%	10%
Percentage to patient service departments	80%	85%	90%

Notes: 1. The allocation percentages are based on a two-year analysis of the actual services provided by the support departments to other departments.

2. To use the percentages to perform an allocation, they may have to be adjusted to ensure that the entire amount of the cost pool is allocated. To illustrate, in the direct method, all of Administration's costs ($500,000) have to be allocated directly in a single allocation to the three patient service departments. If the raw percentages were used, only 35% + 20% + 25% = 80% of the cost pool would be allocated, so the allocation percentages have to be adjusted so that 80 percent represents the entire allocation (100 percent). Thus, instead of a 35 percent allocation to Adult Medicine, its adjusted allocation is 35%/80% = 43.75%. In a similar manner, the adjusted allocation to Obstetrics is 20%/80% = 25%, while the adjusted allocation to Pediatrics is 25%/80% = 31.25%. When done correctly, the adjusted percentages must sum to 100%: 43.75% + 25% + 31.25% = 100%.

EXHIBIT 4.3
Apple Valley Family Practice: Sensitivity Analysis Values

Sensitivity to Changes in Relative Overhead Costs:

New Direct Expenses for Calculation 1

Administration	$4,400,000
Facilities	1,000,000
Finance	1,800,000
Total overhead expenses	$7,200,000

New Direct Expenses for Calculation 2

Administration	$1,000,000
Facilities	1,800,000
Finance	4,400,000
Total overhead expenses	$7,200,000

Sensitivity to Allocation Percentages:

	Percentage of Services Provided By		
Services Provided to	*Administration*	*Facilities*	*Finance*
Administration	—	25%	20%
Facilities	30%	—	20
Finance	30	25	—
Adult Medicine	18	32	33
Obstetrics	10	6	17
Pediatrics	12	12	10
Total	100%	100%	100%
Percentage to support departments	60%	50%	40%
Percentage to patient service departments	40%	50%	60%

BLUE POINTE HEALTHCARE
PREMIUM DEVELOPMENT

5

Blue Pointe Healthcare, a regional not-for-profit managed care company headquartered in Hartford, Connecticut, has more than 1 million enrollees in 25 different plans in Connecticut, Maine, Massachusetts, New Hampshire, Rhode Island, and Vermont. It has recently been contacted by a consortium of employers, including such major companies as IBM, GE, and Prudential, regarding its interest in bidding on a managed care (HMO) contract to be offered to the consortium's 75,000 employees located in and around Nashua, New Hampshire.

Blue Pointe's approach to premium development starts with the recognition that the premium received from employers must cover two different categories of expenses: (1) the cost of providing required healthcare services (medical costs) and (2) the costs of administering the plan and establishing reserves (other costs). Reserves, which typically are required by state insurance regulators, are necessary to ensure that funds are available to pay providers when medical costs exceed the amount collected in premium payments. Blue Pointe, as a not-for-profit corporation, does not explicitly include a profit element in its premium. However, the reserve requirement is set sufficiently high so that income from reserve investments is available to fund product expansion and growth. Thus, in effect, a portion of the reserve requirement constitutes profit.

Blue Pointe uses a multistep approach in setting its premiums. First, a base per member per month (PMPM) cost is estimated for each of the plan's covered benefits. When the premiums are initially established for a new subscriber group, the base PMPM costs are usually developed on the basis of historical utilization and cost data. If data are available on the specific subscriber group, as with the consortium contract, these data are used. Otherwise, the base PMPM costs are based on utilization and cost data from one or more proxy groups, which are chosen to match as closely as possible the demographic, utilization, and cost patterns that will be experienced with the new contract. Also, any utilization or cost savings that will result from Blue Pointe's aggressive utilization management program are factored into the premium.

The base PMPM costs then are adjusted to reflect the dollar amount of copayments to providers as well as the estimated impact of copayment and benefit options on utilization and hence medical costs. Copayments, which are an additional source of revenue to the provider panel, reduce Blue Pointe's medical costs and thus lower the consortium's premium. Furthermore, the higher the copayment, the lower the utilization of that service, especially if it is noncritical. Finally, the more restrictive the benefits package, the lower the costs associated with medical services. The end result, after these adjustments are made, is an adjusted PMPM cost for each service. The adjusted PMPM costs are then summed to obtain the total medical PMPM amount.

To estimate the total nonmedical PMPM amount, Blue Pointe typically adds 15 percent to the total medical PMPM amount for administrative costs and 5 percent for reserves. The sum of the total medical and total nonmedical amounts (called the "total PMPM amount") is the per member amount that Blue Pointe must collect from the consortium each month to meet the total costs of serving the healthcare needs of its employees—the subscribers to the plan.

Once the total PMPM amount is calculated, it must be converted into actual premium rates for individuals and families. Using data provided by the consortium, Blue Pointe estimates that 45 percent of subscribers will elect individual coverage, while the remaining 55 percent will choose family coverage. Blue Pointe plans to offer the consortium a two-rate structure, under which employees may elect either single or family coverage. Data from the consortium indicate that family coverage, on average, includes 3.5 individuals, so, all else the same, the premiums for families should be 3.5 times as much as for individuals. However, children typically consume less healthcare services, on a dollar basis, than do adults, so final premiums must reflect such differentials.

Here are the factor rates for obtaining individual and family premium rates:

Single factor: 1.216   Family factor: 3.356

In setting the specific premium rates, Blue Pointe must ensure that the total premiums collected, which would be paid by both the employer and employees, equal the estimated total calculated using the PMPM rate. The 75,000 population that would be served by the contract consists (roughly) of 12,000 individual members and 18,000 families. Thus, 75,000 x Total PMPM amount must equal (12,000 x Single premium) + (18,000 x Family premium).

Exhibit 5.1 contains a partially completed copy of the worksheet that Blue Pointe uses to establish the total PMPM amount and premium rates on any contract. The worksheet provides a relatively easy guide for implementing the procedures described above. Exhibit 5.2 contains the relevant cost and utilization adjustment factors for a variety of service and copayment options. Once the decision has been made on the appropriate service and copay structure, these adjustment factors feed into the calculations in Exhibit 5.1 for each service's medical PMPM amount.

The consortium has furnished Blue Pointe with a significant amount of data concerning its employees' current utilization of healthcare services. The inpatient cost and utilization data for consortium employees are as follows:

Average daily fee-for-service charge $1,400
Utilization ($10 copay)   500 days per year per 1,000 members

Note, however, that a recent survey of New Hampshire hospitals indicates that most managed care contracts call for per diem payments in the range of $1,000–$1,200. Additionally, Blue Pointe's experience with similar employee groups indicates that moderate utilization management would result in 400–450 inpatient days per 1,000 plan members.

Exhibit 5.3 contains current cost and utilization data for other facility services, including skilled nursing care, inpatient mental health care, hospital surgical services, and emergency department care. The utilization and cost data on primary care services for consortium employees are as follows:

Current number of visits ($5 copay)	3.4 per year per member

Blue Pointe routinely pays primary care physicians a capitated amount based on annual costs of $200,000. Blue Pointe assumes that one primary care physician can handle 4,000 patient visits per year. Utilization and cost data for specialist office visits are as follows:

Current number of visits ($0 copay)	1.5 per year per member
Current cost per visit	$92.65

Note that the total PMPM amount shown in Exhibit 5.1 may be modified to reflect anticipated inflation of medical costs. This adjustment is especially critical if the total PMPM premium is based on old cost data. For the most part, the cost data provided in the case can be assumed to be two years old. (Although the data are for last year, the contract will not be in place for yet another year.)

Also, note that the premium calculation in Exhibit 5.1 does not include certain medical services such as routine vision and dental care, chiropractic services, durable medical equipment, out-of-network services, and pharmacy benefits. The consortium specifically requested that the initial premium bid exclude such "rider" services. However, if Blue Pointe is chosen to submit a final premium bid, the consortium will likely request pricing on one or more riders.

Finally, with no guidance from the consortium regarding the level of services desired or the copay structure, Blue Pointe intends to offer three choices to the consortium: low cost, moderate cost, and high cost. Of course, these plans differ in that the low-cost (to the consortium) plan requires higher copays by employees and has more limitations on covered services; the high-cost plan has lower copays and fewer limitations; and the moderate-cost plan falls between the two extremes.

Assume that you have recently joined Blue Pointe Healthcare as a marketing analyst. Your first task is to develop the bid presentation to be made to the consortium. (**Note: The data in this case are for illustrative purposes only and do not reflect current healthcare costs.**)

EXHIBIT 5.1
Blue Pointe Healthcare: Premium Development Worksheet

I. Medical Expenses

	Base PMPM Cost	Copay Adjustment Factors Cost	Utilization	Adjusted PMPM
Facility Services				
Inpatient:				
Acute	$			$
Skilled nursing				
Mental health				
Substance abuse	0.41	1.0000	1.0000	0.41
Surgical procedures				
Emergency department				
Outpatient procedures	3.43	1.0000	1.0000	3.43
Total facilities				_____
Physician Services				
Primary care services				
Specialist services:				
Office visits				
Surgical services	9.00	0.9544	1.0000	8.59
All other services	23.67	0.8659	0.9100	18.65
Total physicians				_____
Total medical PMPM amount				_____

II. Nonmedical Expenses

Administrative

Reserves

Total nonmedical PMPM amount ══════

III. Total Expenses

Total PMPM amount

IV. Premium Rates

	Single	Family
Rate factor	_____	_____
Premium rate	══════	══════

EXHIBIT 5.2
Blue Pointe Healthcare: Cost and Utilization Adjustment Factors

	Patient Copay Amount	Copay Cost Adj. Factor	Copay Utilization Adj. Factor
Facility Services			
Inpatient acute	$ 0	1.0000	1.0000
	100	0.9851	0.9750
	150	0.9777	0.9600
	250	0.9642	0.9200
Skilled nursing	$ 0	1.0000	1.0000
Mental health:			
30-day limit	$ 0	1.0000	0.9524
	100	0.9805	0.9286
	150	0.9707	0.9143
	250	0.9532	0.8762
60-day limit	$ 0	1.0000	1.2000
	100	0.9845	1.1700
	150	0.9768	1.1520
	250	0.9628	1.1040
90-day limit	$ 0	1.0000	1.2500
	100	0.9851	1.2188
	150	0.9777	1.2000
	250	0.9643	1.1500
Surgical procedures	$ 0	1.0000	1.0000
	100	0.9231	1.0000
	150	0.8846	1.0000
	250	0.8077	1.0000
Emergency department	$ 0	1.0857	1.0250
	15	1.0000	1.0000
	25	0.9429	0.9850
	50	0.8000	0.9550

EXHIBIT 5.2 (continued)
Blue Pointe Healthcare: Cost and Utilization Adjustment Factors

	Patient Copay Amount	Copay Cost Adj. Factor	Copay Utilization Adj. Factor
Primary Care Services	$ 0	1.0352	1.0150
	5	1.0000	1.0000
	10	0.9472	0.9800
	15	0.8593	0.9500
	20	0.7713	0.9200
	25	0.6834	0.8900
Specialist Services			
Zero PCP Copay	$ 0	1.0000	1.0000
	5	0.8897	0.9730
	10	0.7795	0.9590
	15	0.6692	0.9450
$10 PCP Copay	$ 0	1.0000	0.9920
	5	0.8897	0.9600
	10	0.7795	0.9460
	15	0.6692	0.9320
$20 PCP Copay	$ 0	1.0000	0.9680
	5	0.8897	0.9360
	10	0.7795	0.9220
	15	0.6692	0.9080

PCP: primary care physician
Note: Blue Pointe uses various incentive systems to control utilization of specialty services. One system requires PCPs to copay for each specialist office visit.

EXHIBIT 5.3
Consortium Employee Utilization and Cost Data: Other Facility Services

Skilled nursing facility care	25.2 days per year per 1,000 members
Current average daily cost	$650
Inpatient mental care ($0 copay)	64.4 days per year per 1,000 members
Current average daily cost	$740
Hospital-based surgery ($0 copay)	41.7 cases per year per 1,000 members
Current costs	$1,800 per case
Emergency department care ($15 copay)	132 visits per year per 1,000 members
Current costs	$250 per visit (see note)

Note: The emergency department cost is the total charge for facility services, some of which would be covered by the $15 copay.

COLUMBIA MEMORIAL HOSPITAL

BREAK-EVEN ANALYSIS

6

COLUMBIA MEMORIAL HOSPITAL, an acute care hospital with 300 beds and 160 staff physicians, is one of 75 hospitals owned and operated by Health Services of America, a for-profit, publicly owned company. Although two other acute care hospitals serve the same population, Columbia historically has been highly profitable because of its well-appointed facilities, fine medical staff, reputation for quality care, and the amount of individual attention it gives to patients. In addition to the standard range of inpatient and outpatient services, Columbia operates an emergency department within the hospital complex and a stand-alone walk-in clinic located across the street from the area's major shopping mall, about two miles from the hospital.

Patients who need immediate care for injuries or illness, be it a nail-gun puncture or a sore throat, are increasingly turning to walk-in clinics (urgent care centers). These clinics aim to fill the gap between the growing shortage of primary care physicians and already crowded (and expensive) emergency departments. Walk-in clinics are staffed by physicians, offer wait times as little as a few minutes, and charge $60 to $200, depending on the procedure. Furthermore, no appointments are necessary and evening and weekend hours are frequently available. Finally, many offer discounts to the uninsured, and for those with coverage, copayments are typically much less than for emergency department visits. Currently, 8,000 of these clinics exist around the country, including about 1,200 affiliated with hospitals.

50   *Cases in Healthcare Finance*

Mike Reynolds, Columbia's chief executive officer (CEO), is concerned about the clinic's overall financial soundness. About ten years ago, all three area hospitals jumped onto the walk-in-clinic bandwagon, and within a short time, there were five such clinics scattered around the city. Now, only three are left, and none of them appears to be a big money maker. Mike wonders if Columbia should continue to operate its clinic or close it down. The clinic is currently handling a patient load of 45 visits per day, but it has the physical capacity to handle many more visits—up to 85 a day. Mike's decision has been complicated by the fact that Rose Daniels, Columbia's marketing director, has been pushing to embark on a new marketing program for the clinic. She believes that an expanded marketing effort aimed at local businesses would bring in the number of new patients needed to make the clinic a financial winner.

Mike has asked Brent Williams, Columbia's chief financial officer, to look into the whole matter of the walk-in clinic. In their meeting, Mike stated that he visualizes three potential outcomes for the clinic: (1) the clinic could be closed; (2) the clinic could continue to operate as is—that is, without expanding its marketing program; or (3) the clinic could continue to operate, but with the expanded marketing effort. As a starting point for the analysis, Brent has collected the most recent historical financial and operating data for the clinic, which are summarized in Exhibit 6.1. In assessing the historical data, Brent noted that one competing clinic had recently (December 2009) closed its doors. Furthermore, a review of several years of financial data revealed that the Columbia clinic does not have a pronounced seasonal utilization pattern.

Next, Brent met several times with the clinic's director. The primary purpose of the meetings was to estimate the additional costs that would have to be borne if clinic volume rose above the current January/February average level of 45 visits per day. Any incremental usage would require additional expenditures for administrative and medical supplies, estimated to be $3.00 per patient visit for medical supplies, such as tongue blades and rubber gloves, and $0.50 per patient visit for administrative supplies, such as file folders and clinical record sheets.

Because of the relatively low volume level, the clinic has purposely been staffed at the bare minimum. In fact, some clinic employees have started to grumble about not being able to do their jobs well because of overwork. Thus, any increase in the number of patient visits would require immediate administrative and medical staff increases. Furthermore, as the number of visits increase, the clinic would have to hire additional staff members. The incremental costs associated with increased volume are summarized in Exhibit 6.2.

In addition, Brent learned that the building is leased on a long-term basis. Columbia could cancel the lease, but the lease contract calls for a cancellation penalty of three months' rent ($37,500) at the current lease rate. Brent was startled to read in the newspaper that Baptist Hospital, Columbia's major competitor, had just bought the city's largest primary care group practice, and Baptist's CEO said that more group practice acquisitions are planned. Brent wondered whether Baptist's actions would influence the decision regarding the clinic's fate.

Finally, Brent met with Rose (Columbia's marketing director) to learn more about the proposed expansion of the clinic's marketing program. The primary focus of the new marketing program would be on occupational health services (OHS). OHS involves providing medical care to local businesses, including physical examinations for managers and employees; treatment of illnesses that occur during work hours; and treatment of work-related injuries, especially those covered by Workers' Comp. Although some of the clinic's current business is OHS related, Rose believes that a strong marketing effort, coupled with specialized OHS record keeping, could bring additional patients to the clinic. The proposed marketing expansion requires a marketing assistant who will run the clinic's OHS program. Additionally, the new marketing program would incur costs for newspaper, radio, TV, and Internet ads as well as for brochures and handouts. The incremental costs associated with the new marketing program are also summarized in Exhibit 6.2. (To learn more about OHS, start at the American College of Occupational and Environmental Medicine website at www.acoem.org.)

With a blank spreadsheet on the screen, Brent began to construct a model that would provide the information needed to help the board make a rational, informed decision. At first, Brent planned to conduct a standard capital budgeting analysis that focused on the profitability of the clinic as measured by net present value or internal rate of return. Then he realized that the expanded marketing program requires no capital investment. He also realized that no valid data are available on the incremental increase in visits that would be generated either by an increasing population base or by the expanded marketing program.

Finally, he remembered that Mike requested that the analysis consider the inherent profitability of the clinic without the expanded marketing program.

With these points in mind, Brent thought that a break-even analysis would be very useful in making the final decision. Specifically, he wanted to develop answers to the following questions posed by Mike:

1. What is the projected profitability of the walk-in clinic for the entire year if volume continues at its current level?
2. How many additional visits per day would be required to break even without the new marketing program?
3. How many additional visits per day would be required to break even assuming that the new marketing program is undertaken?
4. How many additional daily visits would the new program have to bring in to make it worthwhile, regardless of the overall profitability of the clinic?

In addition, Brent wonders if the clinic could "inflate" its way to profitability; that is, if volume remained at its current level, could the clinic be expected to become profitable in, say, five years, solely because of inflationary increases in revenues? Finally, Brent is concerned about whether or not the analysis gave the clinic full credit for its financial contributions to the hospital. Brent does not want to change the spreadsheet at this late date, but he does want to make sure that any additional financial value is at least considered qualitatively. Overall, Brent must consider all relevant factors—both quantitative and qualitative—and come up with a recommendation regarding the future of the clinic.

EXHIBIT 6.1
Columbia Walk-In Clinic: Historical Financial Data

	CY 2009	Jan 2010	Feb 2010	Monthly Averages 2009	Monthly Averages Jan/Feb 2010	Monthly Averages Total
Number of visits	14,522	1,365	1,335	1,210	1,350	1,230
Net revenue	$548,747	$55,028	$54,748	$45,729	$54,888	$47,037
Salaries and wages	$154,250	$13,540	$13,544	$12,854	$13,542	$12,952
Physician fees	192,000	18,000	18,000	16,000	18,000	16,286
Malpractice insurance	31,440	3,215	3,215	2,620	3,215	2,705
Travel and education	5,365	538	665	447	602	469
General insurance	8,112	843	843	676	843	700
Subscriptions	189	0	0	16	0	14
Electricity	11,820	1,124	1,029	985	1,077	998
Water	1,260	135	142	105	139	110
Equipment rental	1,260	105	105	105	105	105
Building lease	155,745	12,500	12,500	12,979	12,500	12,910
Other operating expenses	103,779	8,152	7,923	8,648	8,038	8,561
Total operating expenses	$665,220	$58,152	$57,966	$55,435	$58,059	$55,810
Net profit (loss)	($116,473)	($3,124)	($3,218)	($9,706)	($3,173)	($8,773)
Gross margin (%)	−21.2%	−5.7%	−5.9%	−21.2%	−5.8%	−18.7%

EXHIBIT 6.2
Columbia Walk-In Clinic: Monthly Incremental Cost Data

	\multicolumn{5}{c}{Number of Additional Visits per Day}
	0	1–10	11–20	21–30	31–40
Variable Costs					
Medical supplies			$3.00 per visit		
Administrative supplies			0.50 per visit		
Total variable costs per visit			$3.50 per visit		
Semifixed Costs					
Salaries and wages		$ 4,000	$ 5,000	$ 6,000	$ 7,000
Physician fees		10,000	10,000	10,000	20,000
Total monthly semifixed costs	$ 0	$14,000	$15,000	$16,000	$27,000
Fixed Costs					
Marketing assistant's salary	$ 3,000	$ 3,000	$ 3,000	$ 3,000	$ 3,000
Advertising expenses	4,000	4,000	4,000	4,000	4,000
Total monthly fixed costs	$ 7,000	$ 7,000	$ 7,000	$ 7,000	$ 7,000

PALISADES MENTAL HEALTH CLINIC
VARIANCE ANALYSIS

7

PALISADES MENTAL HEALTH Clinic is a not-for-profit, multidisciplinary mental health provider that offers both inpatient and outpatient services on a full-risk (capitated) basis to members of managed care plans. Its clinical staff consists primarily of psychiatrists, psychologists, psychiatric nurses, social workers, and chemical dependency counselors. Currently, Palisades has major contracts with two large managed care organizations in its service area: Physician Care (PC) and Share Healthplans (SH). Each of these organizations has both commercial and Medicare HMO contracts with Palisades. Thus, in total, there are four separate product lines.

Palisades is partially funded by state and local governments. The agreement with the funding agencies is that funds received will cover overhead and capital expenses. Furthermore, expenses for drugs and other medical and administrative supplies are billed separately to the HMOs at cost. Thus, overhead and supplies expenses are not part of this budget, which means that the analysis focuses on clinical labor expenses. If the assumption is made that other payment mechanisms cover overhead, capital expenses, and supplies at cost, then Palisades's profitability is solely a function of its ability to create revenues that exceed labor costs. Thus, its operating budget focuses on enrollment, per member premiums, utilization, and labor costs.

Exhibit 7.1 contains the assumptions used to prepare Palisades's 2009 operating budget. Note that the four product lines are expected to provide a total of 4,551,000 member-months of revenue during

2009. Also, note that each product line has a different PMPM payment (premium) amount. Exhibit 7.1 also contains expected admission (for inpatients), referral rate (for outpatients), and labor cost and utilization data for each product line. Because of the unique employment arrangements between Palisades and its clinical staff, in which the staff are paid on the basis of the number of patient service units provided, clinical labor costs are virtually all variable, and hence costs are not identified as fixed or variable.

Exhibit 7.2 contains the forecasted 2009 budget. In essence, data from Exhibit 7.1 are used to forecast revenues and costs, both in the aggregate and by product line. Overall, Palisades expected to earn a profit of $419,379 on these product lines in 2009.

During the first quarter of 2009, Palisades's managers noted a higher utilization rate than budgeted. To add to their concern, the monthly enrollment figures supplied by the contracting managed care plans were less than those budgeted. Together, these trends indicated lower revenues and higher per enrollee costs, and hence lower profits, than forecasted in Exhibit 7.2. These concerns were borne out when the first-quarter profits came in under budget. To help stem the adverse trend, Palisades's managers instituted a utilization management system in which all inpatient stays were required to be approved by the clinic's medical director—a senior staff psychiatrist. In addition, Palisades was able to make mid-year changes to its commercial premiums that increased the average premiums for the year.

Unfortunately, the action taken was "too little, too late" to save the year. Exhibit 7.3 contains operating results for 2009, while Exhibit 7.4 contains the realized aggregate and product line P&L (profit and loss) statements. A quick review of Exhibit 7.4 reveals that the signals conveyed by the first-quarter data were indeed correct; although 2009 ended with a profit, the profit was much less than the amount forecasted.

When the results were submitted to Palisades's chief executive officer, Janet Johnson, she grimaced and said, "I knew it was coming, but I did not expect the profit number to be so low." It was immediately apparent to Janet that Palisades could not afford similar results in 2010. She knew that something had to be done, but the best course of action was not clear.

To help plan for next year, Janet asked Palisades's finance and accounting department head, Bob Mitchell, to perform a variance analysis on the data to help identify the problems that led to the poor financial results for 2009. Unfortunately, Bob's area of expertise is dealing with lenders and other capital suppliers, so he passed the assignment on to you, a newly hired financial analyst.

To start the analysis, you created a diagram (Exhibit 7.5) to help understand variance analysis. (Note that this diagram is generic in nature and has not been "customized" for this case.) Furthermore, you recognize that because the volume variance consists of differences in both enrollment and utilization, it is necessary to create two flexible budgets: one flexed (adjusted) for actual enrollment only, and a second one flexed for both actual enrollment and actual utilization. Additionally, to help with the calculations, you jotted down an equation list for calculating variances. (Note that not all of the equations listed are necessarily applicable to this analysis.) This list is contained in Exhibit 7.6.

Of course, both Janet and Bob are more concerned with what the numbers mean than what the numbers are. Therefore, your variance analysis should include a great deal of interpretation along with the numbers. Finally, you would like to use this assignment to help advance your career within the organization, so you are going to go one step further: Offer recommendations for management action along with the numbers and interpretation.

**EXHIBIT 7.1
Palisades Mental
Health Clinic:
2009 Operating
Budget Assumptions**

Expected Enrollment (Member Months)

PC Commercial	3,365,000
PC Medicare	469,000
SH Commercial	502,000
SH Medicare	215,000
Total	4,551,000

Expected Premium Data (per Member per Month)

PC Commercial	$0.70
PC Medicare	0.85
SH Commercial	0.75
SH Medicare	0.80

Expected Labor Data per Admission or Session

	Inpatient		Outpatient	
	# of Hours	Hourly Rate	# of Hours	Hourly Rate
PC Commercial	53.74	$35	1.04	$100
PC Medicare	68.43	35	1.30	100
SH Commercial	47.77	35	1.15	100
SH Medicare	56.86	35	1.14	100

PC: Physician Care; SH: Share Healthplans

EXHIBIT 7.1 (continued) Palisades Mental Health Clinic: 2009 Operating Budget Assumptions

Expected Utilization and Total Labor Cost Data

			Inpatient			Outpatient		
Plan Type	Avg # Members (in 000s)	Admission Rate	Cost per Admission	Total Costs	Referral Rate	Cost per Session	Total Costs	Total
PC:								
Commercial	280.417	3.81	$1,881	$2,009,639	2.00	$104	$58,327	$2,067,966
Medicare	39.083	3.96	2,395	370,671	2.00	130	10,162	380,833
Total	319.500			$2,380,310			$68,489	$2,448,799
SH:								
Commercial	41.833	3.89	$1,672	$ 272,085	2.00	$115	$ 9,622	$ 281,707
Medicare	17.917	4.17	1,990	148,681	2.00	114	4,085	152,766
Total	59.750			$ 420,766			$13,707	$ 434,473
Grand total	379.250			$2,801,076			$82,196	$2,883,272

PC: Physician Care; SH: Share Healthplans

EXHIBIT 7.2
Palisades Mental Health Clinic: 2009 Operating Budget

Expected Product Line and Aggregate Profits

	PC		SH		
	Commercial	Medicare	Commercial	Medicare	Total
Revenue	$2,335,500	$398,650	$376,500	$172,000	$3,302,650
Costs	2,067,964	380,836	281,709	152,763	2,883,271
Profit	$287,536	$17,814	$94,791	$19,237	$419,379
Margin	12.3%	4.5%	25.2%	11.2%	12.7%

EXHIBIT 7.3
Palisades Mental Health Clinic: 2009 Operating Results

Actual Enrollment (Member Months)

PC Commercial	3,073,133
PC Medicare	485,000
SH Commercial	547,105
SH Medicare	257,000
Total	4,362,238

Actual Premium Data (per Member per Month)

PC Commercial	$0.75
PC Medicare	0.85
SH Commercial	0.80
SH Medicare	0.80

Actual Labor Data per Admission or Session

	Inpatient		Outpatient	
	# of Hours	Hourly Rate	# of Hours	Hourly Rate
PC Commercial	47.32	$38	0.95	$109.50
PC Medicare	58.66	38	1.15	109.50
SH Commercial	52.06	33	0.98	95
SH Medicare	84.85	33	2.00	95

EXHIBIT 7.3 (continued) Palisades Mental Health Clinic: 2009 Operating Results

Actual Utilization and Cost Data

Plan Type	Avg # Members (in 000s)	Inpatient			Outpatient			Total
		Admission Rate	Cost per Admission	Total Costs	Referral Rate	Cost per Session	Total Costs	
PC:								
Commercial	256.094	4.33	$1,798	$1,993,782	3.65	$104	$ 97,213	$2,090,996
Medicare	40.417	4.68	2,229	421,615	1.86	126	9,472	431,087
Total	296.511			$2,415,397			$106,685	$2,522,083
SH:								
Commercial	45.592	5.79	$1,718	$ 453,514	3.35	$ 93	$ 14,204	$ 467,719
Medicare	21.417	4.56	2,800	273,448	1.75	190	7,121	280,569
Total	67.009			$ 726,962			$ 21,325	$ 748,288
Grand total	363.520			$3,142,360			$128,011	$3,270,371

Note: These data were generated on a spreadsheet, and hence some rounding differences occur.

EXHIBIT 7.4
Palisades Mental Health Clinic: 2009 Actual P&L Statements

Product Line and Aggregate Profit Results

	PC		SH		
	Commercial	Medicare	Commercial	Medicare	Total
Revenue	$2,304,850	$412,250	$437,684	$205,600	$3,360,384
Costs	2,090,996	431,087	467,719	280,569	3,270,371
Profit	$ 213,584	($ 18,837)	($ 30,035)	($ 74,969)	$ 90,013
Margin	9.3%	(4.6%)	(6.9%)	(36.5%)	2.7%

Note: These data were generated on a spreadsheet, and hence some rounding differences occur.

EXHIBIT 7.5
Variance Analysis Summary

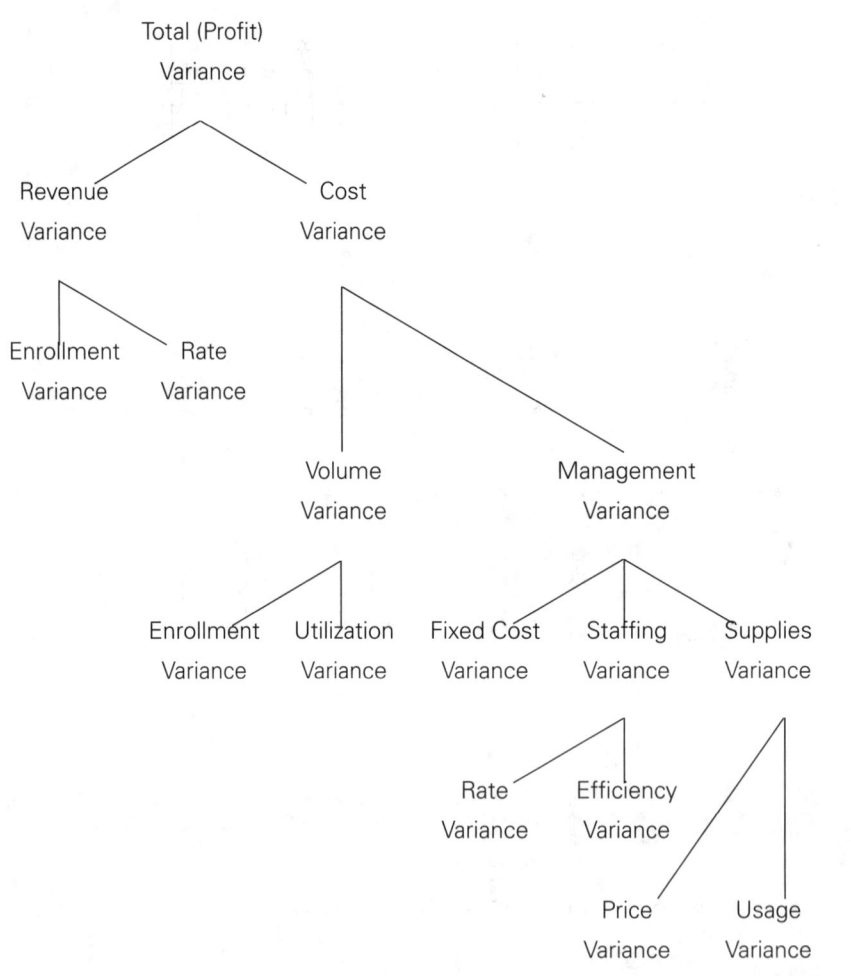

Hint: It might be useful to use this figure as the format for presenting your numerical results.

EXHIBIT 7.6
Generic Equation List

Total variance	= Actual profit − Static profit
Revenue variance	= Actual revenue − Static revenue
Enrollment variance	= Flexible (enrollment) revenue − Static revenue
Rate variance	= Actual revenue − Flexible (enrollment) revenue
Cost variance	= Static costs − Actual costs
Volume variance	= Static costs − Flexible (enrollment/utilization) costs
Enrollment variance	= Static costs − Flexible (enrollment) costs
Utilization variance	= Flexible (enrollment) costs − Flexible (enrollment/utilization) costs
Management variance	= Flexible (enrollment/utilization) costs − Actual costs
Fixed cost variance	= Actual fixed costs − Flexible fixed costs
Staffing variance	= Actual staffing costs − Flexible (enrollment/utilization) staffing costs
Rate variance	= (Static hourly labor rate − Actual hourly labor rate) × Actual number of hours per episode × Actual utilization rate × Actual enrollment
Efficiency variance	= (Expected number of hours per episode − Actual number of hours per episode) × Expected hourly labor rate × Actual utilization rate × Actual enrollment
Supplies variance	= Flexible (enrollment/utilization) supplies costs − Actual supplies costs
Price variance	= (Static price − Actual price) × Actual units
Usage variance	= (Flexible units − Actual units) × Static price

Note: Not all of the above equations are necessarily useful to all product lines.

ALPINE VILLAGE CLINIC

CASH BUDGETING

8

ALPINE VILLAGE CLINIC is a small walk-in clinic located next to the primary ski area of Alpine Village, a winter resort close to Aspen, Colorado. The clinic specializes in treating injuries sustained while skiing. It is owned and operated by two physicians: James Peterson, an orthopedist, and Amanda Cook, an internist. The clinic has an outside accountant who takes care of payroll matters, but Dr. Cook does all the other financial work for the clinic. However, to help in that task, the clinic recently hired a part-time MBA student, Doug Washington.

On a Wednesday afternoon in October 2009, Dr. Cook called Doug into her office to tell him that she had just received a phone call from the head of commercial lending at First Bank of Aspen, the clinic's primary lender. Because of a forecasted reduction in bank deposits and hence funds available to make commercial loans, First Bank has asked each of its commercial loan customers for an estimate of its borrowing requirements for the first half of 2010.

Dr. Cook had a previously scheduled meeting at First Bank the following Monday to discuss cash management services, so she asked Doug to come up with an estimate of the clinic's line-of-credit requirements to submit at the meeting. A line of credit is a short-term loan agreement by which a bank agrees to lend a business some specified maximum amount. The business can borrow (draw down) against the credit line at any time it is in force, which typically is no longer than one year. When a line expires, it will have to be renegotiated if it is still needed. The amount borrowed on the line, or some lesser amount, can be repaid at any time, but any amount outstanding must be repaid at expiration. Interest is charged daily on the amount drawn down, and often a commitment fee is required up front to secure the line. In general, lines of credit are used by businesses to meet temporary (usually seasonal) cash needs, as opposed to being used for permanent long-term financing.

Dr. Cook was going on vacation, a trip that had already been delayed several times, and she would not be back until just before her meeting at the bank. Therefore, she asked Doug to prepare a cash budget while she was away. No one had taken the time to prepare a cash budget recently, although a spreadsheet model that had been constructed a few years ago was available for use. From information previously developed, Doug knew that no seasonal financing would be needed from First Bank before January, so he decided to restrict his budget to the period from January through June 2010. As a first step, he looked through the clinic's financial records to get the data needed to develop the billings forecast, which is contained in Exhibit 8.1.

Patient volume at the clinic is highly seasonal because the vast majority of the business occurs during the ski season, which generally runs from December through March. In fact, at one time Dr. Peterson and Dr. Cook thought about closing the clinic during the slow months. However, (1) the clinic would be very difficult to operate efficiently for only a portion of the year, and (2) the area has started to attract a sizable number of summer visitors, which has made summer operations more financially attractive.

On the basis of the clinic's previous collections experience, Doug was able to convert billings for medical services into actual cash collections. On average, about 20 percent of the clinic's patients pay immediately for services rendered. Third-party payers pay the remaining claims, with 20 percent of the payments made within 30 days and the 60 percent remainder (of total billings) paid within 60 days. For monthly budgeting purposes, 20 percent of billings are assumed to be collected in the month of billing, 20 percent are assumed to be collected one month after the billing month, and 60 percent are assumed to be collected two months after the billing month.

Variable medical costs at the clinic are assumed to consist entirely of medical and administrative supplies. These supplies, which are estimated to cost 15 percent of billings, are purchased two months before expected usage. On average, the clinic pays about half of its suppliers in the month of purchase (two months before use) and the other half in the following month (one month before use).

Clinical labor costs (for physicians and other clinical employees) are the primary expense of the clinic. During the high season (December through March), these costs run $150,000 a month, but some of the clinical staff work only seasonally, so clinical labor costs drop to $120,000 a month in the remaining months.

The clinic pays fixed general and administrative expenses, including clerical labor, of approximately $30,000 a month, while lease obligations amount to $12,000 per month. These expenditures are expected to continue at the same level throughout the forecast period. The clinic's miscellaneous expenses are estimated to be $10,000 monthly.

The clinic has a semi-annual, five-year, 10 percent, $500,000 term loan outstanding with First Bank. Payments of $64,752 are due on March 15 and September 15. Also, the clinic is planning to replace an old x-ray machine (which has no salvage value) in February with a new one that costs $125,000. The clinic is a partnership, so, for tax purposes, any profits (or losses) are prorated to the two physician partners, who must pay individual taxes on this income. Thus, no tax payments are built into the clinic's cash budget.

The clinic has to maintain a minimum cash balance of $50,000 at First Bank because of compensating balance requirements on its term loan. This amount, but no more, is expected to be on hand on January 1, 2010.

If a daily cash budget is required, some additional assumptions about volume and collections are required:

1. The clinic operates seven days a week.
2. Patient volume is more or less constant throughout the month, so the daily billings forecast will be 1/(Number of days in the month) multiplied by the billings forecast for that month.
3. Daily billings follow the 20 percent, 20 percent, 60 percent collection breakdown based on monthly billings.
4. Patient payments are assumed to occur on the day of billing, "early" payers are assumed to pay 30 days after billing, and "late" payers are assumed to pay 60 days after billing.

5. The lease payment is made on the 1st of the month.
6. Fifty percent of both clinical labor costs and general and administrative expenses are paid on the 1st of the month, and 50 percent are paid on the 15th of the month.
7. Supplies are delivered on the 1st of the month and paid for on the 5th of the month.
8. Miscellaneous expenses are incurred and paid evenly throughout each month.
9. Term loan payments are made on the 15th of the month in which they are due.
10. The compensating balance of $50,000 must be in the bank on each day.

In addition to the cash budget itself, Dr. Cook asked Doug to consider several additional issues:

1. Will the clinic need to request a line of credit for the period and, if so, how big should the line be?
2. A monthly budget may not reveal the full extent of the borrowing requirements actually needed. To see if her concern is valid, Dr. Cook suggested that Doug construct a daily cash budget for the month of January as a test case.
3. The existing cash budget model does not provide for interest paid on line-of-credit borrowings or interest earned on cash surpluses. Dr. Cook suggested that the monthly cash budget be modified to include these items. Currently, the interest rate on First Bank line-of-credit draw downs is 8 percent compounded monthly (8%/12 = 0.667% per month), and First Bank pays 4 percent compounded monthly (4%/12 = 0.333% per month) on temporary investments of excess cash.
4. Although the target cash balance has been based on First Bank's compensating balance requirement, the term loan will be paid off in September 2010. Dr. Cook asked how the clinic might go about setting its target cash balance when no compensating balance is required.

5. Dr. Cook is well aware that the cash budget is a forecast, so most of the cash flows shown are expected values rather than amounts known with certainty. If actual patient billings, and hence collections, were different from forecasted levels, then the forecasted surpluses and deficits would be incorrect. Dr. Cook is interested in knowing how various changes in key assumptions would affect the forecasted surplus or deficit. For example, if billings fell below the forecasted level or if collections were stretched out, what effect would that have?
6. Dr. Cook notes that no bad-debt losses are built into the budget. How would that be accomplished if the clinic had such losses?
7. Finally, Dr. Cook believes that the surge in patient volume over the forecast period is bound to result in some cash surpluses, and she wants to know what the clinic should do with them.

Place yourself in Doug's position. Be prepared to discuss your analysis with Dr. Cook when you meet with her next week.

EXHIBIT 8.1
Alpine Village Clinic: Billings Forecast

Year	Month	Amount
2009	November	$150,000
	December	250,000
2010	January	350,000
	February	450,000
	March	300,000
	April	150,000
	May	100,000
	June	175,000
	July	250,000
	August	200,000

BOSTON TRANSPLANT CENTER

MARGINAL COST PRICING ANALYSIS

BOSTON TRANSPLANT CENTER (the Center), which is part of University Healthcare System, is a regional leader in the intense and medically sophisticated area of organ transplants. All transplants are performed at Boston General Hospital, the 400-bed flagship of the System.

Craig MacLeod, the director of the Center, has been at the job for ten years, during which time significant growth has occurred in both the number of transplant programs and the volume of procedures performed. When Craig joined the Center he was put in charge of a kidney transplant program that was averaging 60 transplants per year and a heart transplant program that was performing 40 transplants per year. Today, the Center performs more than 500 transplants annually, including transplants from liver, lung, and pancreas programs.

The liver transplant program is the most successful of all organ programs in terms of volume and revenues. Last year, volume totaled 120 transplants, bringing in more than $50 million in total revenues. This year Craig is optimistic that the liver program can do even better. However, he knows that increased volume is largely dependent on the number of organ donors and his success in negotiating a new managed care contract with the Transplant Management Corporation (TMC), the largest transplant-benefits company in the nation.

Although most health insurers can identify those patients who are good candidates for transplant services, only the largest health insurers have the expertise to manage the transplant process. The reason is that transplants are relatively rare in comparison with other, more conventional medical procedures. However, the costs to insurers for transplant services are typically high—usually in the six- or seven-figure range. To ensure the best and most cost-effective management of transplant services, most insurers outsource transplant management to companies, such as TMC, that specialize in these services.

Contracting for transplant services is unique and complex because of the sophistication of the medical procedures involved. Transplant services consist of five phases: (1) patient evaluation, (2) patient care while awaiting surgery, (3) organ procurement, (4) surgery and the attendant inpatient stay, and (5) one year of follow-up visits. The costs involved in Phase 1 are relatively simple to estimate, but the remaining phases can be extremely variable in terms of resource utilization, and hence costs, because of differences in patient acuity and surgical outcomes.

Historically, reimbursement for transplant services has been handled in a number of different ways. Initially, many transplant providers bundled all five phases together and offered insurers a single, global rate. Although this method simplified the contracting process, the rate set was often chosen on the basis of building market share rather than on covering costs. Indeed, many institutions could not even estimate with any confidence the true costs of providing transplant services.

Somewhat ironically, success in gaining market share usually increases the financial risk of the transplant program because higher volumes increase the likelihood of higher acuity patients. Furthermore, changes in the organ allocation system have promoted the acceptance of sicker patients into transplant programs. Although the total costs associated with all phases of a liver transplant average about $400,000, the amount can more than quadruple if the patient requires a re-transplant or if other complications occur. Because of this extreme variability in costs, outlier protection is a critical aspect of contract negotiations if the reimbursement methodology is a fixed prospective rate such as a global rate.

The TMC contract requires the approval of Dr. Armand Lee, the newly appointed surgical director of the liver transplant program. Fortunately, Dr. Lee shared Craig's enthusiasm to build the liver program into one of the largest in the country and, like Craig, was motivated to secure the contract. In his second meeting with Dr. Lee, Craig discussed the specifics of the current contract negotiations. Phases 1, 2, and 5 will be reimbursed at a set discount from charges. Furthermore, to reduce the amount of financial risk borne by the Center, Phase 3 (organ procurement) will be reimbursed on a cost basis. This makes sense because the cost of Phase 3 is almost completely uncontrollable by the Center. Thus, the primary focus of the negotiations, and the make-or-break part of the contract, is the reimbursement amount for Phase 4. (For more information on organ procurement, see the United Network for Organ Sharing website at www.unos.org.)

Phase 4 costs are divided into two categories: hospital costs and physician costs. Physician reimbursement has already been agreed on, with TMC agreeing to pay a fixed amount per physician work relative value unit (WRVU). Thus, the primary matter at hand involves hospital costs. To aid in the negotiations, Craig compiled the Phase 4 hospital costs of the last 12 liver-transplant patients. These data are presented in Exhibit 9.1.

When Dr. Lee read the numbers, he was amazed. A total average cost of $119,805 for 19 days average length of stay translates to a per diem average cost of more than $6,000. He was sure that TMC would not be willing to sign a contract that paid the hospital $120,000 (or more) to cover Phase 4 costs. Thus, Dr. Lee suggested that Craig reexamine the cost structure to see if these costs could be reduced.

At first glance, it appeared to Craig that a large cost savings could be realized by merely reducing the average length of stay (LOS). For example, it appeared that Phase 4 hospital costs associated with a particular patient could be reduced by over $12,000 by merely reducing the LOS by two days. However, further analysis revealed the costs associated with Phase 4 are not a linear function of LOS. Internal studies at the Center indicated that the first day of Phase 4 is usually the most costly while the last day is usually the least costly. Indeed, roughly 70 percent of Phase 4 costs occur in the first 24 hours of hospitalization.

When it appeared that it would be difficult to lower Phase 4 hospital costs, Craig decided to pursue a different strategy. He believed that economies of scale are present in liver transplants, and hence the marginal cost of each transplant is lower than the average cost. Thus, Craig proposed basing the Phase 4 hospital reimbursement amount on marginal rather than total (full) costs.

Assume that you have been hired as a consultant to recommend a fixed reimbursement amount (the base rate) that should be proposed in the contract negotiations for Phase 4 hospital services. To help in the analysis, Craig has indicated that approximately 60 percent of nursing, ancillary, operating room, and laboratory costs are fixed. The remaining costs—radiology, drug, and other services—are predominantly variable. Furthermore, current payers are reimbursing the hospital at roughly $140,000 for these services, and there is sufficient capacity to handle about 30 more transplants before fixed costs will increase by a meaningful amount.

In addition, you have been asked to recommend a method for handling outliers, including the threshold amount and additional reimbursement scheme. Other programs within the Center use two methods for outlier payments. One method is to charge an additional per diem amount based on an LOS threshold. Alternatively, some percentage of costs above the base rate can be charged when a cost threshold is reached. (For more information on how Medicare treats outliers, go to www.cms.hhs.gov and then search "inpatient outliers.")

As you think about the problem at hand, several questions come to mind. First, would it be useful to identify the underlying cost structure of the Phase 4 hospital services? (It might help in thinking about the relevant issues.) Second, should the hospital worry about a long-term pricing strategy, or is it sufficient to think in terms of the first year contract only? Finally, if the price is set significantly less than the average reimbursement amount paid by current payers, what impact would that have on future negotiations with those payers?

EXHIBIT 9.1
Boston Transplant Center: Phase 4 Hospital Costs (millions of dollars)

Patient	Age	LOS	Total Costs	Nursing Cost	Ancillary Cost	OR Cost	Lab Cost	Radiology Cost	Drug Costs	Other Costs
A	61	25	$141,092	$10,261	$65,416	$6,770	$13,712	$1,483	$20,992	$22,458
B	56	15	139,306	11,969	63,668	8,501	7,409	2,261	24,504	20,994
C	42	12	74,259	6,939	33,661	3,128	5,279	668	6,964	17,620
D	52	13	115,349	7,221	54,063	5,779	6,112	903	7,638	33,633
E	12	26	172,613	28,205	72,204	6,847	10,550	1,766	23,061	29,980
F	59	22	83,807	16,858	33,474	4,654	6,211	1,397	9,698	11,515
G	41	25	136,060	9,645	63,208	6,489	13,091	1,382	20,127	22,118
H	35	17	139,308	11,969	63,669	8,501	7,409	2,261	24,505	20,994
I	52	12	74,259	6,939	33,660	3,128	5,280	668	6,964	17,620
J	38	13	115,348	7,221	54,063	5,778	6,111	903	7,639	33,633
K	59	25	166,224	26,909	69,657	6,765	10,061	1,677	22,007	29,148
L	60	21	80,034	15,629	32,202	4,531	5,937	1,293	9,122	11,320
Average	47	19	$119,805	$13,314	$53,245	$5,906	$8,097	$1,389	$15,268	$22,586

LOS: length of stay; OR: operating room

DENVER HEALTH NETWORK

ABC ANALYSIS

10

DENVER HEALTH NETWORK (the Network), a newly created subsidiary of Denver Health System (the System), consists of five medical group practices. When initially acquired, the practices were placed in a for-profit subsidiary, but concerns over both Stark Law provisions and the fact that the practices were barely profitable prompted the System to place them in the newly created not-for-profit subsidiary.

The practices include both primary care and specialty physicians, with an emphasis on obstetrics/gynecology, surgery, pediatrics, and psychology. Although the physicians are administratively organized into five groups, they practice at only three different locations, each one staffed with a physician mix of primary care and specialists. In spite of the fact that its direct contribution to system profitability is negligible, the Network is considered an essential part of the System because it generates a large amount of indirect income from both inpatient referrals and the use of outpatient ancillary services. In fact, it has been estimated that each dollar of revenue generated by the Network leads to $8 of inpatient and ancillary revenues. By limiting the amount of ancillary services provided at the Network locations, patients are forced (or at least encouraged) to use other System facilities for such services.

Still, some ancillary services are best performed at the Network locations for one or more of the following reasons: lower costs, increased physician efficiency, and improved patient convenience. For example, one of the practice locations has a diagnostic imaging capability. When the scanner was moved from another facility to the Network location, volume increased, costs decreased, and both physician and patient satisfaction improved.

The Network is considering a proposal to provide ultrasound services at its locations. Preliminary analysis indicates that two approaches are most suitable. Alternative 1 involves the purchase of one ultrasound machine for each of the Network's three locations. Patients would schedule appointments, generally at the clinic that they are using, during preset times on particular days of the week. Then, the full-time ultrasound technician would travel from one location to another to administer the tests as scheduled.

In Alternative 2, patient scheduling would be the same, but only one ultrasound machine would be purchased. The machine would be mounted in a van that the technician would drive to each of the three Network locations. Most of the operating costs of the two alternatives are identical, but Alternative 2 has the added cost of operating the van and setting up the machine after each move.

The two alternatives differ substantially in capital investment costs because Alternative 1 requires three ultrasound machines, at a cost of $100,000 each, while Alternative 2 requires only one. However, Alternative 2 requires a van, which with necessary modifications would cost $40,000. Thus, the capital costs for Alternative 1 total 3 × $100,000 = $300,000, while those for Alternative 2 amount to only $100,000 + $40,000 = $140,000.

Note, though, that because the two alternatives have different operating costs, a proper cost analysis of the two alternatives must include both capital investment and operating costs. The Network financial staff, which in reality is the System financial staff, considered several methods for estimating the operating costs of each alternative. After much discussion, the chief financial officer (CFO) decided that the activity based costing (ABC) method would be best. Furthermore, an ad hoc task force was formed to perform the cost analysis.

To begin the ABC analysis, the task force had to develop the activities involved in the two alternatives. This was accomplished by conducting "walk-throughs" of the entire process from the standpoints of the patient, the ultrasound technician, and the billing and collections department. The results are contained in Exhibit 10.1. A review of the activities confirms that all except one—transportation and setup—are applicable to both alternatives.

The next step in the ABC process is to detail the costs associated with each activity. This step uses financial, operational, and volume data, along with the appropriate cost driver for each activity, to estimate resource consumption. Note that traditional costing, which often focuses on department-level costs, typically first deals with direct costs and then allocates indirect (overhead) costs proportionally according to a predetermined allocation rate. In ABC costing, the activities required to produce some service, including both direct and indirect, are estimated simultaneously. For example, Exhibit 10.1 contains activities that entail direct costs (such as technician time) and activities that entail indirect costs (such as billing and collection). Although the ABC method is more complex and hence costlier than the traditional method, it is the only way to accurately (more or less) estimate the costs of individual services.

Activity cost detail on a per procedure basis is contained in Exhibit 10.2. In essence, each activity is assigned a cost driver that is most highly correlated with the actual utilization of resources. Then the number of driver units, along with the cost per unit, is estimated for each activity. The product of the number of units and the cost per unit gives the cost of each activity. Finally, the activity costs are summed to obtain the total per procedure cost.

Many of the activity costs cannot be estimated without approximating the number of ultrasounds that will be performed. The best estimate is that 50 procedures will be done each week, regardless of which alternative is chosen. Assuming the technician works 48 weeks per year, the annual volume estimate is 2,400 procedures. Of course, one factor that complicates the analysis is that a much greater total volume can be accommodated under Alternative 1, with three machines, than with Alternative 2, with only one machine. However, to keep the initial analysis manageable, the decision was made to assume the same annual volume regardless of the alternative chosen.

In addition to the costs mentioned thus far, some other costs are thought to be relevant to the decision. First, in addition to the obvious costs of operating the van (primarily gas expenses), annual maintenance costs will run about $1,000. Furthermore, annual maintenance costs on each of the three machines under Alternative 1 are estimated at $500, while the annual maintenance costs for the single machine under Alternative 2 are estimated at $1,000 because of added wear and tear. Also, the manufacturer of the ultrasound machines has indicated that a discount may be available if three machines, as opposed to only one, are purchased. The amount of the discount is somewhat uncertain, although 5 percent has been mentioned.

Finally, to have a rough estimate of total annual costs over the life of the equipment, it is necessary to make assumptions about the useful life of the ultrasound machines and the van. Although somewhat controversial, the decision was made to assume a five-year life for both the ultrasound machines and the van. Furthermore, the assumption was made that the value of these assets would be negligible at the end of five years.

Assume that you are the chairperson of the ad hoc task force. Your charge is to evaluate the two alternatives and then make a recommendation on which one to accept, assuming that revenues would be identical for the two alternatives, and hence the decision can be made solely on the basis of costs. As part of the analysis, it will be necessary to estimate the costs of the two alternatives on a per procedure and annual basis. In addition, any qualitative factors that are relevant to the decision must be considered before the recommendation is made.

To keep the analysis manageable, the task force was instructed to assume that operating costs remain constant over the useful life of the equipment. For comparative purposes, this assumption is not too egregious because the activities are roughly the same for both alternatives, and hence inflation would have a somewhat neutral impact on costs.

In addition to the base case analysis, the System CFO has asked the task force to perform some sensitivity (scenario) analyses. First, he is concerned about the accuracy of the cost detail inputs. Although there is some confidence in many of the estimates, others are more arbitrary. Those activity cost inputs that are considered to be most uncertain are supplies cost per unit, billing and collection cost per unit, general administration cost per unit, and transportation and setup cost per unit. Thus, the task force has been asked to redo the analysis assuming that these inputs are higher than the base case values by 10 percent and 20 percent. Activity cost inputs that are less than the base case values can also be examined, but the critical issue here is not to underestimate the total costs involved in the two alternatives.

Along the same lines, the task force also has to figure out what would happen to the cost estimates if the useful life of the capital equipment is as short as three years or as long as seven years. Another concern is that the useful life of the equipment depends on the alternative chosen; that is, Alternative 1 presents less wear and tear than Alternative 2. Finally, the task force has to assess the impact of the purchase discount—would a higher discount amount influence the ultimate decision?

Although you believe that it is useful to perform a sensitivity analysis on the number of procedures, doing so requires recalculation of the per unit cost inputs, which may be too time consuming to undertake at this point in the analysis.

EXHIBIT 10.1
Denver Health Network: Activities Associated with Alternatives 1 and 2

1. Appointment scheduling
2. Patient check-in
3. Ultrasound testing
4. Patient check-out
5. Film processing
6. Film reading
7. Billing and collection
8. General administration
9. Transportation and setup (Alternative 2 only)

EXHIBIT 10.2
Denver Health Network: Activity Cost Detail

Activity	Cost Driver	Volume	Cost per Unit
Appointment scheduling	Receptionist time	3 minutes	$ 0.20
Patient check-in	Receptionist time	5 minutes	0.20
Ultrasound testing	Technician time	45 minutes	0.40
	Physician time	1.5 minutes	3.00
	Supplies	per procedure	9.00
Patient check-out	Receptionist time	5 minutes	0.20
Film processing	Technician time	10 minutes	0.40
Film reading	Contract terms	per procedure	40.00
Billing and collection	Overhead costs	per procedure	6.80
General administration	Overhead costs	per procedure	1.25
Transportation and setup	Technician time	6 minutes	1.00

Notes:
1. Physician time for testing (15 minutes) is needed for one of every ten patients.
2. Supplies consist of linen, probe cover, gel, film, and print paper.
3. There are no radiologists in the Network. Films will be read by the Hospital's radiologists at a contract fee of $40 per procedure.
4. Billing and collection costs are based on an average cost per medical services bill.
5. General administration costs are based on an estimate of facilities and other administrative costs.
6. Transportation and setup is based on ten procedures per day at each location and includes vehicle operating costs, excluding maintenance.

MAITLAND FAMILY PHYSICIANS

11

PAY FOR PERFORMANCE

MAITLAND FAMILY PHYSICIANS is a medical group practice located in Maitland, Maine. The practice has four family practice physicians and a medical support staff consisting of a practice manager, two receptionists, four nurses, two medical assistants, two billing clerks, and one laboratory technician. Data relevant to the practice are contained in Exhibits 11.1 through 11.3.

The practice is organized as a partnership, with each physician having an equal share. Although the practice manager has the authority to make the day-to-day business decisions, all strategic decisions regarding the management of the practice are made jointly by the partners. In addition, the practice uses a local accountant (CPA) to prepare and file its taxes and to act as a financial advisor when needed.

The current policy of the practice is to provide equal compensation to the physicians. Last year, each physician was paid the same monthly salary ($12,500) and then, at the end of each year, profits of the practice that were not needed for reinvestment in new assets were divided equally among the partners ($30,000 each). This policy of "equal pay for equal work" has been in place since the practice was founded in 1996, but discontentment is growing among the partners regarding this compensation system. Not surprisingly, each of the physicians believes that he or she is working harder than the others and hence should receive greater compensation. In addition, the physicians have recognized that it is important to start putting away some profits to pay for new medical equipment to replace aging items as well as to expand the range of services offered.

A recent survey by the Medical Group Management Association indicated that less than 10 percent of group practice family physicians are compensated on a straight salary basis, while the majority is compensated on the basis of productivity. Of those compensated on the basis of productivity, about half are paid solely on that basis while half receive a base salary plus a bonus component based either on productivity exclusively or on productivity plus other measures. (For more information on the Medical Group Management Association, see www.mgma.com.)

In an effort to reward those physicians who are truly working harder as well as to create the incentive for all physicians to be as productive as possible, the partners directed the practice manager to assess the current compensation system and to recommend any changes that would improve the system.

Assume that you are the practice manager of Maitland Family Physicians. As a start, you scheduled a meeting with the partners to develop some initial guidance. At this meeting, the partners agreed that any proposed system must have the following five characteristics:

1. *The system must be **trusted**.* Physicians must trust not only the data used but also the integrity and competency of the individuals who administer the system. The compensation model itself may be sound, but a lack of faith in either the data or the administration of the system will lead to a lack of confidence in the entire system.

2. *The system must be clearly **understood**.* In the search for the perfect system, it is easy to create a model that is too complex, and hence the links between pay and performance cannot be easily identified. If the physicians cannot easily identify what performance is necessary to increase pay, the system will not have the desired results.

3. *The system must be perceived to be **equitable**.* If the physicians do not believe that the system is fair—that is, those physicians who contribute more are paid more—then the system is doomed to fail.

4. *The system must create the proper **incentives**.* A fundamental objective of any compensation plan is to

maintain the financial viability of the organization. Thus, the model must create incentives that promote behavior that contributes to the success of the group. Furthermore, the incentives offered must be large enough to encourage physicians to change behavior.

5. *The system must be **affordable***. The costs of implementing and administering the system must be reasonable. Furthermore, the total amount of incentive compensation paid must not impair the ability of the practice to cover its operating costs, replace existing assets, or acquire new assets.

The general agreement among the physicians was that the compensation system should consist of a base salary plus some form of pay for performance. For example, each physician might receive a base salary of $6,000 per month with the remaining compensation based on some measure(s) of performance.

Even with this agreement, the task of making recommendations for change in the physician compensation system seemed daunting. After all, many systems are available, and each system has its own strengths and weaknesses. To gain a better appreciation of the possible choices, you download from the Internet several articles about pay for performance and meet with the group's accountant (Jennifer Wong) to learn about the alternative systems being used at other practices. After several meetings with Jennifer, you conclude that several potential measures may be appropriate for Maitland's pay for performance plan.

Productivity measures:
- *Number of patient visits.* This measure is a simple count of the annual number of patient visits for a physician, regardless of the time per visit, type of visit, or reimbursement amount. More patient visits indicate higher physician productivity.
- *Work RVUs.* Jennifer consulted with another group practice that uses Relative Value Units (RVUs) to measure productivity. RVUs form the basis of physician compensation for Medicare services. Under this system, each physician service has three relative

value components: (1) physician work, (2) practice expense, and (3) malpractice expense. More work RVUs indicate higher productivity.
- *Professional procedures.* This measure is a simple count of the annual number of procedure codes (such as injections), regardless of the time per procedure, type of procedure, or reimbursement amount. More professional procedures indicate higher productivity.

Financial measures:
- *Gross charges.* This measure is the total gross charges generated by a physician during the year (discounts, allowances, and costs are ignored). Gross charges are easily identified from the current billing system used by the practice. A greater amount of gross charges indicates higher physician financial performance.
- *Net collections.* This measure is the total collected revenue generated by a physician during the year (gross charges minus discounts and allowances, but costs are again ignored). Net collections are also easily identified from the current billing system used by the practice. A greater amount of net collections indicates higher financial performance.
- *Net income.* This measure is the total net income (before physician compensation) generated by a physician during the year. As stated above, gross charges and net collections are easily identified from the current billing system used by the practice. However, this measure requires allocation of practice costs to individual physicians. With limited data at hand, one possible solution is to divide the total costs of the practice into fixed and variable components, then allocate the fixed component equally to all four physicians and allocate the variable component on the basis of some measure of resource utilization, such as professional procedures. A greater amount of net income indicates higher financial performance.

Quality measures:
- *Average patient satisfaction.* This measure is an average of the patient satisfaction scores for a physician. Greater patient satisfaction indicates higher physician quality.
- *Blood pressure control.* This measure indicates whether or not a physician met a target for blood pressure control among the patients seen during the year. The Center for Medicare & Medicaid Services (CMS) is currently sponsoring the Physician Group Practice (PGP) Demonstration Project (see www.cms.hhs.gov/DemoProjectsEvalRpts/downloads/PGP_Demo_Design.pdf). Participating physicians are eligible to earn separate quality payments if they meet performance targets on a variety of quality measures. Blood pressure control is one of the quality measures that apply to all Medicare beneficiaries who meet age and sex criteria. Attaining the target indicates higher quality.
- *Breast cancer screening target met.* This is another PGP Demonstration Project quality measure that applies to all Medicare beneficiaries who meet age and sex criteria. Attaining the target indicates higher quality.

Of course, any combination of the above measures could also be used, so a wide variety of solutions is possible.

Armed with the above information, you held another meeting with the partners (and Jennifer Wong) to gain some additional insights into their views regarding physician compensation. The meeting had three agenda items:

1. Should pay for performance be based on productivity, financial performance, and/or quality?
2. What total dollar amount should be allocated to performance pay versus base salary?
3. What amount of net income (after physician compensation) should the group target?

At the beginning of the meeting, all agreed that the physicians who contribute most to the practice should receive the highest compensation. However, it soon became clear that no agreement exists on how to define "contribute most." For example, one physician stated that work effort is the most meaningful measure. "Let's just use the number of patient visits—it's simple and we all agree that more visits require more work," he argued. But this was challenged by another physician who stated that many of her patients were elderly and chronically ill who require much more time per visit than younger, healthier patients. Work RVUs would be another basis of measuring productivity, but the physicians were not sure about using data from a billing system for such a purpose.

Another physician argued that the real money is in procedures. Historically, physicians have been paid relatively well for diagnostic and treatment procedures and group practices that do a lot of procedures have done well financially. Therefore, it made sense to consider rewarding those physicians who performed higher numbers of professional procedures. But another physician was uncomfortable with rewarding such a narrow part of clinical practice. "Besides," he said, "I am getting older and don't do as many procedures as I once did."

The discussion then turned to financial performance measures. Although one physician strongly believed that gross charges were the best measure, another countered that (1) gross charges do not reflect reimbursement amounts, and (2) gross charges generated at the expense of high costs do not help the group much financially. Jennifer jumped in at that point saying that the strength of the net income measure is that physicians are held responsible for both revenues and costs. Thus, physicians would have the incentive to be both more productive (generate more revenues) and, at the same time, reduce the costs associated with operating the practice. However, the cost allocation required for calculation of net income can only be roughly accomplished, so it will be difficult to convince the physicians that the allocation has true economic meaning.

Performance pay based on quality was the last item discussed. One physician stated that there is too much emphasis on money. If the physicians do not provide high quality medical care and keep their patients happy, there will be no patients and hence no revenues. Thus, she argued, "patient satisfaction is just as important as revenue generation." In addition to the patient satisfaction issue, one partner noted that Maitland physicians provide care to many Medicare beneficiaries. "It's important to gain experience with the pay for quality approach that CMS is supporting," he argued. However, the reaction to this comment was mixed. Two partners thought the whole idea of rewarding physicians for practicing good medicine was ludicrous. One commented that the profession is in a sad state of affairs if physicians have to be paid extra to do what is right. On the other hand, another partner stated that if this was the trend among payers, it may be wise to consider building similar quality guidelines into Maitland's compensation system.

At the end of the discussion on Agenda Item 1, one physician stated, "It's clear we don't agree on how to measure performance, so why don't we just use all of the measures? Then everybody will be happy." The thought of using all of the measures made you shudder because of the complexity of interpreting the results and the administrative burden required.

Then, the meeting turned to Agenda Item 2: the actual amount to be allocated to performance pay. One physician suggested that because no agreement was reached on how to measure performance, most compensation should be base salary and only a small amount should be allocated for performance pay—say $10,000 per physician. This brought a chorus of "why bother" from the other physicians. "This isn't enough of an incentive for anything—after all, we spend more than that on lattes," one joked. In contrast, another physician stated, "I'd prefer to base all of our compensation on performance. Who can argue with productivity, financial performance, and quality?" After a prolonged discussion, the only agreement reached was that the dollar amount allocated to performance pay should be enough to make physicians pay attention to it but should be less than the amount allocated for base salary.

Agenda Item 3 revolved around the target net income (after physician compensation). In contrast to the other agenda items, all of the physicians readily agreed that the net income after physician compensation of the practice had to be at least $70,000 to pay for new medical equipment that the practice requires.

At the end of the meeting, you could tell that the job would not be an easy one. None of the approaches that were initially identified could be ruled out. Furthermore, there was only broad direction on the dollar amount to be allocated for performance pay. Your major hurdle would be to develop a system that would be supported by all four partners. Thus, the ability to "sell" the system to the partners is just as important as the system itself.

To ensure an orderly approach to the assignment, you decide to (1) use the historical allocation between base salary and performance pay as a starting point, (2) assess the sensitivity of physician pay to the various performance measures, and (3) recommend the system that you believe is best for Maitland Family Physicians. Finally, you recognize that the merits of alternative compensation systems are influenced somewhat by the nature of the practice's revenue stream (reimbursement). Almost half of the practice's revenues come from Medicare and Medicaid, while the remainder comes from commercial insurers, including managed care plans. Although some of the managed care plans were using capitated payment systems several years ago, all of the practice's payers now use fee-for-service methodologies.

EXHIBIT 11.1
Maitland Family Physicians: Historical Support Staff Salaries

	Number of Employees	Total Compensation
Practice manager	1	$ 75,168
Receptionists	2	48,652
Nurses	4	175,264
Medical assistants	2	52,615
Billing clerks	2	62,165
Laboratory technician	1	46,788
Other costs		61,736
Total		$522,388

Note: Other costs include accounting fees and other fees for outsourced services.

Gross charges		$2,242,648
Net collections		$1,747,059
Practice expenses:		
Support staff salaries	$ 522,388	
Facilities cost	298,351	
Supplies cost	136,257	
Total practice expenses		$ 956,996
Net income before physician compensation		$ 790,063
Physician compensation:		
Base salaries	$ 600,000	
Bonus	120,000	
Total physician compensation		$ 720,000
Net income after physician compensation		$ 70,063

EXHIBIT 11.2 Maitland Family Physicians: Historical Financial Data

	Physician Identifier				
	A	B	C	D	Total
Patients visits	4,023	3,567	3,966	4,244	15,800
Number of RVUs	4,667	5,055	5,475	4,967	20,164
Professional procedures	6,255	6,972	7,287	6,742	27,256
Gross charges	$527,820	$535,841	$602,675	$567,312	$2,242,648
Net collections	$422,256	$401,881	$421,872	$501,050	$1,747,059
Average patient satisfaction score	89	80	87	94	
Blood pressure control target met?	Yes	Yes	Yes	No	
Breast cancer screening target met?	No	Yes	No	No	

RVUs: relative value units

Notes: 1. The RVUs listed are work RVUs, which are only one of the three components used in Medicare physician reimbursement.
    2. Over the past five years, the average annual amount reinvested in the practice was $65,000.
    3. Patient satisfaction scores are on a scale of 100.

EXHIBIT 11.3 Maitland Family Physicians: Historical Physician Data

Financial Management Basics

PENSACOLA SURGERY CENTERS

12

TIME VALUE ANALYSIS

GARY HUDSON was born and raised in Pensacola, Florida. He obtained his bachelor's degree in business from Florida State University, where he enrolled in the NROTC program, and, after graduation, he received a commission in the U.S. Marine Corps. After his release from active duty, Gary used his GI Bill benefits to obtain a master's degree in health services administration from the University of Florida. His first job in healthcare was as a special projects coordinator/financial analyst at a large Miami hospital. He enjoyed his work there, but his ultimate goal was to return to Pensacola as the manager of a smaller healthcare business, where he would have more responsibility and authority. After five years in Miami, Gary became the chief operating and financial officer of Pensacola Surgery Centers, an investor-owned chain of ambulatory surgery centers with six locations in the panhandle area of Florida.

Immediately after assuming his new position, Gary found himself facing several decisions. First, the company currently has $100,000 in its cash account, but its target cash balance is only $50,000. Thus, Gary wants to temporarily invest the excess $50,000 in marketable securities, which typically consist of low-risk, short-term securities, such as Treasury bills or money market mutual funds. One alternative Gary is considering is to invest the $50,000 in a bank certificate of deposit (CD). CDs are generally available in maturities from six months to ten years, and interest can be handled in one of two ways: the investor (buyer) can receive periodic interest payments or the interest can automatically be reinvested in the CD. In the latter case, the buyer receives no interest during the life of the CD but receives the accumulated interest plus principal amount at maturity. Because the goal of this investment is to accumulate funds for future use, as opposed to generate current income, all interest earned on the CD will be reinvested.

Second, the company recently bought a new hardware/software system to handle its patient billings. However, the current system obviously will have to be replaced with a more sophisticated system in about five years. After making some inquiries to potential vendors, Gary estimated the future cost of the new system to be $200,000. To ensure that the funds are available to make this purchase, Gary is planning either to deposit a lump sum today in an interest-bearing account or to make annual payments into the same account.

Third, Pensacola Surgery Centers has some extra space at one of its locations that it might lease out for five years. The initial renovation cost, which includes new flooring and lighting as well as a new outside entrance, is estimated to be $40,000. Because of some unusual terms in the proposed lease contract, and also because of a promise to add more computer ports in three years, the net cash inflows expected from the lease follow this uneven pattern:

End of Year	Net Cash Flow
1	$ 12,000
2	14,000
3	2,000
4	16,000
5	20,000

The decisions that Gary faces all involve time value analysis. As a check on your skills, see if you can answer the following relevant questions:

1. Consider the $50,000 excess cash. Assume that Gary invests the funds in a one-year CD.
    a. What is the CD's value at maturity (future value) if it pays 10 percent (annual) interest?

b. What will its future value be if the CD pays 5 percent interest? If it pays 15 percent interest?
c. BankSouth offers CDs with 10 percent nominal (stated) interest, but compounded semiannually. What is the effective annual rate on this CD? What will the future value be after one year if $50,000 were invested?
d. The Pensacola branch of Bank of America offers a 10 percent CD with daily compounding. What are the CD's effective annual rate and its value at maturity one year from now if $50,000 is invested? (Assume a 365-day year.)
e. What stated rate will BankSouth have to offer to make its semiannual-compounding CD competitive with Bank of America's daily-compounding CD?

2. Rework Parts a through d of Question 1 assuming that each CD has a five-year maturity.

3. Now consider the surgery centers' goal of having $200,000 available in five years to buy a new patient billing system.
a. What lump sum amount must be invested today in a CD paying 10 percent annual interest to accumulate the needed $200,000?
b. What annual interest rate is needed to produce $200,000 after five years if only $100,000 is invested?

4. Now consider a second alternative for accumulating funds to buy the new billing system. In lieu of a lump sum investment, assume that five annual payments of $32,000 are made at the end of each year.
a. What type of annuity is this?
b. What is the present value of this annuity if the opportunity cost rate is 10 percent annually? 10 percent compounded semiannually?
c. What is the future value of this annuity if the payments are invested in an account that pays 10 percent interest annually? 10 percent compounded semiannually?

d. What annual interest rate is required to accumulate the $200,000 needed to make the purchase, assuming a $32,000 annual payment?
e. What size annual payment is needed to accumulate $200,000 under annual compounding at a 10 percent interest rate?
f. Suppose the payments are only $16,000 each, but they are made every six months, starting six months from now. What will the future value be if the ten payments were invested at 10 percent annual interest? If invested at BankSouth at 10 percent compounded semiannually?

5. Assume now that the payments are made at the beginning of each period. Repeat the analysis in Question 4.

6. Now consider the uneven cash flow stream stemming from the lease agreement given in the case.
   a. What is the present (Year 0) value of the annual lease cash flows if the opportunity cost rate is 10 percent annually?
   b. What is the future value of this cash flow stream at the end of Year 5 if the cash flows are invested at 10 percent annually? What is the present value of this future value when discounted at 10 percent? What does this result indicate about the consistency inherent in time value analyses?
   c. Does the office renovation and subsequent lease agreement appear to be a good investment for the company? (Hint: Compare the cost of renovation with the present value of the lease payments. Use a 10 percent discount rate for the analysis.)

7. Now assume that it is five years later and the company is unable to accumulate the $200,000 needed to make the software purchase. Instead, it is forced to borrow the $200,000. The loan calls for repayment in equal annual installments over a four-year period, with the first payment due at the end of one year. Assuming that the company can borrow the funds at a 10 percent rate, what amount of interest and principal will be repaid at the end of each year of the loan?

8. Throughout this case, you have been either discounting or compounding cash flows. Many financial analyses, such as bond refunding decisions, capital investment decisions, and lease decisions, involve discounting projected future cash flows. What is the appropriate rate in such situations? What factors influence the value of this rate?

SOUTHEASTERN SPECIALTY, INC.

13

FINANCIAL RISK

SOUTHEASTERN SPECIALTY, INC. (SSI), is a not-for-profit corporation formed by physicians in the College of Medicine at Southeastern University. SSI, with more than 600 physicians, provides the medical staff for University Hospital. In addition, SSI staffs and administers a network of 25 ambulatory care clinics and centers at ten locations within 50 miles of the hospital. In 2009, SSI generated more than $500 million in revenues from about 40,000 inpatient stays and 750,000 outpatient visits.

More than 70 percent of SSI's revenues come from inpatient stays, but this percentage has been declining, and by 2014, more than half of SSI's revenues are expected to stem from outpatient services. As improvements are made in technology and third-party payers continue to pressure providers to cut costs, more and more inpatient services will be converted to outpatient and home care. For example, in 1999, 80 percent of SSI's ophthalmological surgeries took place in University Hospital, while in 2009, 80 percent were conducted in outpatient settings.

Although SSI has traditionally provided only specialty services, in 2004 it instituted a "personal physician services" program, in which patients can receive both primary and specialty care from College of Medicine physicians. This was the first step in SSI's drive to develop an integrated delivery system, which offers a full range of patient services. Now that the system is in place, SSI is contracting with managed care plans to provide virtually all physician services required locally by plan members. Furthermore, SSI is examining the feasibility of contracting directly with employers and hence bypassing managed care plans, but no decision has yet been made. Indeed, state insurance industry representatives expressed opposition to the idea when SSI first announced the possibility of direct contracting. The insurance industry position is that direct contracting with employers to provide a complete healthcare benefit package is an insurance function, which can be undertaken only by licensed insurance plans.

As part of its continuing education program, SSI holds monthly "nonclinical grand rounds" for its physicians, in which various staff members and outside specialists conduct seminars on nonclinical topics of interest. As part of this series, Chris Johnson, SSI's chief financial officer, has been invited to conduct two sessions on the financial risk inherent in integrated delivery systems. His main concern is that physicians, although very sophisticated in clinical matters, have a very limited understanding of basic financial risk concepts and will not appreciate the financial issues involved in integrated delivery systems without first gaining an understanding of basic financial risk concepts. Thus, he plans to devote the entire first session to basic concepts.

In preparation for the seminar, Chris developed the return distributions for the five investments shown in Exhibit 13.1. To create the table, he first hypothesized that five economic states are possible for the coming year, ranging from poor to excellent. Next, he estimated the one-year returns on each investment under each state. The five investments are (1) T-bills, (2) real asset investment Project A, (3) real asset investment Project B, (4) an index fund designed to proxy the returns on the Standard & Poor (S&P) 500 stock index, and (5) an equity investment in SSI itself. T-bills are short-term (one year or less maturity) U.S. Treasury debt securities; Project A is a proposed sports medicine clinic; and Project B is a Medicaid-funded project for providing family health services to an underserved area. Note that Chris developed the returns for Projects A and B and for SSI as a whole by assessing the impact of each economic state on healthcare utilization and reimbursement patterns.

In addition to the returns on these alternative investments, Chris developed the following questions to use as the structure for his presentation. See if you can answer them.

1. Is the return on the one-year T-bill risk free?
2. Calculate the expected rate of return on each of the five investment alternatives listed in Exhibit 13.1. Based

solely on expected returns, which of the potential investments appears best?

3. Now calculate the standard deviations and coefficients of variation of returns for the five alternatives. (Hint: Coefficient of variation of return is defined as the standard deviation divided by the expected rate of return. It is a standardized measure of risk that assesses risk per unit of return.)
   a. What type of risk do these statistics measure?
   b. Is the standard deviation or the coefficient of variation the better measure?
   c. How do the five investment alternatives compare when risk is considered?

4. Suppose SSI forms a two-asset portfolio by investing in both Projects A and B.
   a. To begin, assume that the required investment is the same for both projects—say, $5 million each.
      (1) What will be the portfolio's expected rate of return, standard deviation, and coefficient of variation?
      (2) How do these values compare with the corresponding values for the individual projects?
      (3) What characteristic of the two return distributions makes risk reduction possible?
   b. What do you think will happen to the portfolio's expected rate of return and standard deviation if the portfolio contained 75 percent of Project A? If it contained 75 percent of Project B?

5. Now consider a portfolio that consists of investments in Project A and the S&P 500 Fund.
   a. First, consider a portfolio containing equal investment in the two assets. Will this portfolio have the same risk-reducing effect as the Project A/Project B portfolio considered in Question 4? Explain.
   b. What are the expected returns and standard deviations for a portfolio mix of 0 percent Project A, 10 percent Project A, 20 percent Project A, and so on—up to 100 percent Project A?

6. Suppose an individual investor starts with a portfolio that consists of one randomly selected stock.

a. What will happen to the portfolio's risk if more and more randomly selected stocks are added?
b. What are the implications for investors? Do portfolio effects have an impact on the way investors should think about the riskiness of individual securities?
c. Explain the differences between stand-alone risk, diversifiable risk, and portfolio risk.
d. Suppose that you choose to hold a single stock investment in isolation. Should you expect to be compensated for all of the risk that you assume?

7. Now change Exhibit 13.1 by crossing out the state of the economy and probability columns and replacing them with Year 1, Year 2, Year 3, Year 4, and Year 5. In other words, assume that the distributions represent historical returns earned on each asset in each of the last five years.
   a. Plot four lines on a scatter diagram (regression lines) that show the returns on the S&P 500 Fund (the market) on the x-axis and (1) T-bill returns, (2) Project A returns, (3) Project B returns, and (4) SSI returns on the y-axis.
      (1) What are these lines called?
      (2) Estimate the slope coefficient of each line. What is the slope coefficient called, and what is its significance? (If you have a calculator with statistical functions or are using a spreadsheet, use linear regression to find the slope coefficients.)
      (3) What is the significance of the distance between the plot points and the regression line—that is, the errors?
   b. Plot two lines on a different scatter diagram that show the returns on SSI (the company) on the x-axis and (1) Project A returns and (2) Project B returns on the y-axis.
      (1) What are these lines called?
      (2) Estimate the slope coefficient of each line. What is the slope coefficient called, and what

is its significance? (If you have a calculator with statistical functions or are using a spreadsheet, use linear regression to find the slope coefficients.)

c. If you were an individual investor who could buy any of the assets in Exhibit 13.1, which one(s) would you buy? Why? (Hint: To help answer this question, construct a Security Market Line graph and plot the expected returns on each asset on the graph. Also, note that SSI is actually a not-for-profit corporation, so it is impossible to buy an equity interest in the company. For this question, assume that SSI is an investor-owned company.)

d. Now assume that you are the chief executive officer of SSI and you have to decide whether to invest in Project A, Project B, or both. Which project(s) would you choose if you could accept both? If you could only accept one of the two, which would you choose? Why? (Hint: To help answer this question, construct a "Corporate Market Line" graph, which plots corporate betas rather than market betas on the x-axis, and plot the expected returns for each project on the graph.)

8. a. What is the market risk of each project (A and B) relative to the aggregate market risk of SSI? (For this question, assume that SSI is an investor-owned company.) No additional calculations are necessary.

b. What is the corporate risk of each project (A and B) relative to the aggregate corporate risk of SSI? No additional calculations are necessary.

9. a. What is the efficient markets hypothesis (EMH)?

b. What impact does this theory have on decisions concerning investments in securities?

c. Is the EMH applicable to real asset investments, such as the decision of SSI to invest in Project A or Project B?

d. What impact does the EMH have on corporate financing decisions?

EXHIBIT 13.1
Southeastern Specialty, Inc.: Estimated One-Year Return Distributions on Five Investments

State of the Economy	Probability	Estimated Return on Investment				
		1-Year T-Bill	Project A	Project B	S&P 500 Fund	Equity in SSI
Poor	0.10	7.0%	−8.0%	18.0%	−15.0%	0.0%
Below average	0.20	7.0	2.0	23.0	0.0	5.0
Average	0.40	7.0	14.0	7.0	15.0	10.0
Above average	0.20	7.0	25.0	−3.0	30.0	15.0
Excellent	0.10	7.0	33.0	2.0	45.0	20.0

Note: These return distributions are fictitious and not meant to describe actual market conditions at the time you work this case.

ATLANTIC HEALTHCARE (A)
BOND VALUATION

14

ATLANTIC HEALTHCARE IS an investor-owned hospital chain that owns and operates nine hospitals in Maryland, Virginia, and the District of Columbia. Marcia Long, a recent graduate of a prominent health administration program, has just been hired by Washington Medical Center, Atlantic's largest hospital. Like all new management personnel, Marcia must undergo three months of intensive indoctrination at the system level before joining the hospital.

Marcia began her indoctrination in January 2010. Her first assignment at Atlantic was to review its latest annual report. This was a stroke of luck for Marcia because her father owned several bonds issued by Atlantic, and Marcia was especially interested in whether or not her father had made a good investment. To glean more information about the bonds, Marcia examined Note E to Atlantic's consolidated financial statements, which lists the company's long-term debt obligations, including its first mortgage bonds, installment contracts, and term loans. Exhibit 14.1 contains information on three of the first mortgage bonds listed in Atlantic's annual report. (For more information on bond ratings, see Standard & Poor's website at www.standardpoor.com or the Moody's Investors Services website at www.moodys.com.)

Unfortunately, Atlantic's chief financial officer, Hugo Welsh, found out about Marcia's interest in the firm's debt financing. "Because you are so interested in our financial structure," he said, "here are some questions that I've developed as part of a debt financing presentation to our executive committee. See if you can answer them."

Marcia viewed Hugo's questions as a challenge, as she was convinced that she knew as much about debt financing as most finance MBAs. Apparently Marcia was right because she answered the questions with no difficulty. In fact, Hugo was so impressed that he asked Marcia to give the presentation to the executive committee, which turned out to be a big success.

See if you can do as good a job as Marcia in answering the following questions:

1. To begin, refer to the three bonds listed in Exhibit 14.1. Note that each bond matures at the end of the listed year, and the remaining term to maturity is also listed in the exhibit. Furthermore, each bond has a $1,000 par value, each had a 30-year maturity when it was issued, and all three bonds currently have a 10 percent required nominal rate of return.
   a. Why do the bonds' coupon rates vary so widely?
   b. What would be the value of each bond if it had annual coupon payments?
   c. Atlantic's bonds, like virtually all bonds, actually pay interest semiannually. What is each bond's value under these conditions? Are the bonds currently selling at a discount or at a premium?
   d. What is the effective annual rate of return implied by the values obtained in Part c?
   e. Would you expect a semiannual payment bond to sell at a higher or lower price than an otherwise equivalent annual payment bond? Look at the values calculated in Parts b and c for the five-year bond. Are the prices shown consistent with your expectations? Explain.
2. Now, regardless of your answers to Question 1, assume that on January 1, 2010, the 5-year bond is selling for $800.00, the 15-year bond is selling for $865.49, and the 25-year bond is selling for $1,220.00. (Use these same prices, and assume semiannual coupons, for all of the remaining questions in this case.)
   a. What is the stated (as opposed to effective annual) yield to maturity (YTM) on each bond? (Note: The stated rate is also called the nominal rate.)

b. What is the effective annual YTM on each issue?
c. In comparing bond yields with the yields on other securities, should the stated or effective YTM be used? In comparing yields among bonds, should the stated or effective YTM be used? Explain.
d. Explain the economic meaning of YTM.
3. Suppose Atlantic has a second bond with 25 years left to maturity (in addition to the one listed in Exhibit 14.1) that has a coupon rate of 7 3/8 percent and a January 1, 2010, market price of $747.48.
   a. What are (1) the stated and (2) the effective annual YTMs on this bond?
   b. What is the current yield on each of the 25-year bonds?
   c. What is each of the 25-year bonds' expected price on January 1, 2011, and its capital gains yield for 2010, assuming no change in interest rates? (Hint: Remember that the nominal YTM on each 25-year bond, which is assumed to be its required rate of return, is 10.18 percent.)
   d. What will happen to the value (and price in an efficient market) of each 25-year bond over time? (Again, assume constant future interest rates.)
   e. What is the expected total (percentage) return on each 25-year bond during 2010?
   f. If you were a tax-paying investor, which of the two 25-year bonds would you prefer? Why? What impact will this preference have on the prices, and hence YTMs, of the two bonds?
4. Consider the riskiness of the three bonds listed in Exhibit 14.1.
   a. Explain the difference between price risk and reinvestment rate risk.
   b. Which of the bonds has the most price risk? Why?
   c. Assume that you bought 5-year, 15-year, and 25-year bonds, all with a 10 percent coupon rate and semiannual coupons, at their $1,000 par values. Which bond's value will be affected most if interest rates rise to 13 percent? Which will be affected least?

d. Assume that your investment horizon (or expected holding period) is 25 years. Which of the bonds listed in Exhibit 14.1 has the greatest reinvestment rate risk? Why? Is there a type of bond you could buy to eliminate reinvestment rate risk?
e. Assume that you plan to keep your money invested, and to reinvest all interest receipts, for five years. Furthermore, assume you bought the five-year bond for $800, and interest rates suddenly fell to 5 percent and remained at that level for five years.
   (1) Set up a timeline that can be used to calculate the actual (realized) rate of return on the bond. (Hint: Each interest receipt must be compounded to the maturity date at the reinvestment rate and then summed, along with the maturity value. Then, the rate of return that equates this terminal value to the initial price of the bond is the bond's realized rate of return.) How does your answer compare with the bond's YTM?
   (2) What if interest rates had risen to 15 percent rather than fallen to 5 percent?
   (3) How would the results have differed if you had bought the 25-year bond rather than the 5-year bond?
f. Today, many bond-market participants are speculators as opposed to long-term investors. If you thought interest rates were going to fall from current levels, what bond maturity would you buy to maximize short-term capital gains?
5. Now assume that the 15-year bond is callable after five years at $1,050.
   a. What is its yield to call (YTC)? (Hint: Set up the cash flows on a timeline. If the bond is called, investors will receive interest payments for five years and then receive $1,050 [$1,000 in principal and call premium of $50] at the end of five years. The YTM on this cash flow stream is the bond's YTC.)

b. Do you think it is likely that the bond will be called? Explain.
6. Discuss the basic differences between the bonds issued by investor-owned corporations and those issued by not-for-profit healthcare organizations through municipal financing authorities.
7. Explain how investors set required rates of return on debt securities. (Hint: Think in terms of the real risk-free rate plus any risk borne by investors.)
8. What is the term structure of interest rates? What is a yield curve? Why is the yield curve important to both investors and managers?
9. Briefly describe the bond rating system, including the names of the major rating agencies, the ratings used, the criteria for assigning ratings, and the importance of ratings to both investors and managers. Also, describe the concept of credit enhancement and how issuers should evaluate whether or not to use it.

Face Amount	Coupon Rate	Maturity Date	Years to Maturity	S&P Bond Rating
$ 48,000,000	4 1/2	12/31/14	5	A+
32,000,000	8 1/4	12/31/24	15	A+
100,000,000	12 5/8	12/31/34	25	A+

EXHIBIT 14.1
Atlantic Healthcare:
Partial Long-Term Bond Listing

ATLANTIC HEALTHCARE (B)
STOCK VALUATION

15

ATLANTIC HEALTHCARE is an investor-owned hospital chain that owns and operates nine hospitals in Maryland, Virginia, and the District of Columbia. Marcia Long, a recent graduate of a prominent health services administration program, has just been hired by Washington Medical Center, Atlantic's largest hospital. Like all new management personnel, Marcia must undergo three months of intensive indoctrination at the system level before joining the hospital.

In Case 14, Atlantic Healthcare (A), Marcia conducted an analysis of the firm's bonds and presented her findings to the company's executive committee. Atlantic's chief financial officer, Hugo Welsh, was quite impressed with the quality of Marcia's presentation. Furthermore, the other members of the committee stated that they learned a great deal about debt financing from Marcia's presentation and that they would like to see a similar presentation on equity financing. Because Marcia would be leaving corporate headquarters to start her hospital assignment in less than four weeks, Hugo immediately assigned her the task of analyzing the firm's equity situation and preparing another presentation for the executive committee.

Marcia began by reexamining the firm's annual report to get some basic data. Then, she searched the *Wall Street Journal*, *Value Line*, and other potential sources of financial data to obtain some market data as well as analysts' forecasts for the firm. Exhibit 15.1 contains the information that Marcia developed. (Information on thousands of stocks, including beta estimates, can be obtained from websites such as Yahoo finance (http://finance.yahoo.com), CNN/Money (http://money.cnn.com), Bloomberg (http://bloomberg.com), and MSN Money (http://moneycentral.msn.com).

As in Case 14, Hugo did not want Marcia to go off on a tangent, so he provided her with a list of questions to answer. Also as before, Marcia welcomed the challenge of working on a task traditionally assigned to finance MBAs rather than to graduates of health services administration programs. Put yourself in Marcia's shoes and see how you would fare if assigned this task and needed to answer the following questions:

1. a. What are Atlantic's historical earnings and dividend growth rates over the entire 2004–2009 period? (Hint: Use 2004 data for the present values; 2009 data for the future values, and 1 as the number of periods.)
   b. What are the average annual compounded growth rates? (Hint: Use 2004 data for the present values, 2009 data for future values, and 5 as the number of periods.)
   c. Which rate (overall or annual) better expresses the concept of growth?
2. a. What is the firm's payout ratio in 2009? (Hint: The payout ratio is the percentage of earnings paid out to stockholders as dividends.)
   b. What is Atlantic's average payout over the past six years?
   c. If the payout ratio of an average investor-owned hospital company were about 50 percent, is Atlantic's payout about average, below average, or above average? What is the primary factor that influences a business's payout ratio?
3. a. What is the Capital Asset Pricing Model? What is the Security Market Line (SML)?
   b. Graph the SML using the data presented in Exhibit 15.1.
   c. What would happen to the SML if investors' risk aversion increased and the required rate of return on the market rose to 12 percent?

d. Return to the base case data in Part b of this question. What would happen to the SML if inflation expectations increased by 1 percentage point? (Hint: Investors would add 1 percentage point to their required rates of return on all assets, including risk-free assets.)
e. Return to the base case data in Part b of this question. According to the SML, what is the required rate of return on Atlantic's stock? Plot that point on your SML graph.

4. For now, disregard the dividend growth rates given in Exhibit 15.1. Assume that analysts estimated that Atlantic will have a long-term (constant) dividend growth rate of 5.0 percent. Furthermore, Exhibit 15.1 gives a 2009 dividend (D_0) of $0.48 and an end-of-year (December 31, 2009, or January 1, 2010) stock price (P_0) of $8.00.
   a. What is the expected rate of return on Atlantic's stock if it is purchased on January 1, 2010?
   b. What is the expected dividend yield and expected capital gains yield?
   c. What is the relationship between dividend yield and capital gains yield over time under constant growth assumptions?
   d. What conditions must hold to use the constant growth model? Do many real-world stocks satisfy the constant growth assumptions?
   e. Plot the expected rate of return found in Part a on the SML graph from Question 3. Based on the data developed so far, would you buy Atlantic's stock?

5. Now consider the fact that Value Line predicted that Atlantic's dividends will grow at a 10 percent rate for the next five years and the growth rate will fall to a steady state (constant) 4 percent into the foreseeable future.
   a. Under these conditions, what is the value of Atlantic's stock at the beginning of 2010? (Hint: Lay out the expected dividends on a timeline up to

and including the first year of constant [4 percent] growth. Use the expected dividend in Year 6 and the constant growth model to calculate the value of the stock at the end of Year 5. Discount this Year 5 value, along with the dividends expected in Years 1–5, back to Year 0. Sum these present values to obtain the value of the stock. Dividends are paid at the end of the year.)

  b. Assume that the value you calculated is the actual stock price on January 1, 2010. What is the expected stock price at the end of 2010 assuming that the stock is in equilibrium? At the end of 2011, 2012, 2013, and 2014?

  c. What are the expected dividend yield, capital gains yield, and total return for 2010, 2011, 2012, 2013, and 2014?

6. Atlantic's stock price is $8.00 at the beginning of 2010. Using the growth rates given in Exhibit 15.1 (and also used in Question 5), what is the stock's expected rate of return? (Hint: This is not an easy question. A model similar to the one used to answer Question 5 must be applied, but a trial-and-error technique must be used to find the discount rate that discounts the expected dividend [and Year 5 stock value] stream back to the current price, $8.00. The process is complicated by the fact that each discount rate selected in the trial-and-error process must be used to find the Year 5 stock value before it is used to discount the expected cash flow stream back to Year 0.)

7. What is the efficient markets hypothesis, and what are its implications for stock investors?

EXHIBIT 15.1
Atlantic Healthcare: Selected Stock Data

Historical Data:

Year	Earnings per Share	Dividends per Share
2004	$1.14	$0.21
2005	1.32	0.32
2006	1.54	0.35
2007	1.56	0.36
2008	1.80	0.39
2009	2.00	0.48

Assumed Current (January 1, 2010) Data:

Current stock price	$8.00
Estimated dividend growth rates:	
Next 5 years	10.0%
Long-term steady state	4.0%
Market data:	
Yield on long-term Treasury bonds	5.0%
Merrill Lynch estimate of market returns	11.0%
Value Line beta coefficient	1.2

*Capital
Acquisition*

SOUTHERN HOMECARE
COST OF CAPITAL

16

Southern Homecare was founded in 1992 in Miami, Florida, as a taxable partnership by Maria Gonzalez, MD; Ramon Garcia, RN; and Ron Sparks, LPT. Its purpose was to provide an at-home alternative to hospitals and ambulatory care facilities for basic healthcare services provided by physicians, registered nurses, licensed practical nurses, and physical therapists. (For more information on home health services, see the website of the National Association for Home Care & Hospice at www.nahc.org.)

The partnership enjoyed enormous success in the beginning. Even its founders were surprised at how easy the business was to establish and run. Formation of the company coincided with the search by third-party payers for alternative, and potentially less costly, delivery settings. On the basis of its success in metropolitan Miami, the partnership expanded services into Fort Lauderdale and West Palm Beach and then moved into other metropolitan areas in Florida and across the Southeast. The partnership also expanded services at each location to include occupational, speech, and rehabilitation therapies.

The founders had sufficient personal resources to start the company, and they had enough confidence in their business plan to commit most of their own funds to the new venture. However, after only six years, the external capital requirements brought on by rapid growth exhausted their personal funds, and they were forced to borrow heavily. Soon, although they still needed external capital to finance growth, the founders' ability to borrow at reasonable rates was exhausted. Thus, in 2002 they incorporated the partnership, and in 2005 they sold common stock to the public through an initial public offering (IPO). The founders still retain a large, but minority, ownership position in the company, and currently the stock trades in the over-the-counter market.

Southern is widely recognized as one of the regional leaders in its industry, and it won an award in 2008 for being one of the 100 best-managed small companies in the United States. The company has two operating divisions: (1) the Healthcare Services Division and (2) the Information Systems Division. The Healthcare Services Division operates Southern's home health care services in 22 locations. Because sales and earnings in this division are relatively predictable, the division's business risk is about average.

The Information Systems Division sells the computer software system that Southern designed to control its own operations to other home health care companies. This system combines inventory control, visit scheduling, clinical record keeping, billing and collections, and payroll into a single integrated package. Although the system is excellent, this division competes head to head with several major software firms as well as with information services and management consulting firms. Because of this competition, and the rapid technological changes inherent in the information services field, Southern's management considers the Information Systems Division to have more business risk than the Healthcare Services Division.

Although the company's growth was exceptional, it was more random than planned. The founders simply decided on a location for a new office, ran an advertisement in a local newspaper to recruit clinical professionals and clerical employees, sent in an experienced manager from one of the established offices, and began to make money almost immediately. Formal decision structures were almost nonexistent, but the company's head start and its bright, energetic founders easily overcame any deficiencies in managerial decision-making processes.

However, recent changes in the market for home health care services portend a much more difficult environment in the future. First, relatively generous payment amounts in the 1990s and most of the 2000s produced intense competition in the home health care industry. Other investor-owned home health care firms sprang up like weeds, especially in major cities, and several hospitals in Southern's service area, including not-for-profits, began to offer home health care services.

Second, the rapid increase in expenditures on home health care services prompted payers to drastically reduce reimbursement amounts, just as new capacity came on line. In particular, the Balanced Budget Act of 1997 mandated lower payment amounts for Medicare home health services, which resulted in a totally new prospective payment system (PPS). (For more information on PPS, see www.cms.hhs.gov/center/hha.asp.)

Because of these changes, Southern's board of directors concluded that the company must start to apply state-of-the-art techniques in both its operations and its corporate managerial processes. As a first step, the board directed the financial vice president (VP) to develop an estimate for the company's cost of capital. The financial VP, in turn, directed Southern's treasurer, Clark Ruffin, to prepare and submit a cost-of-capital estimate in two weeks.

Clark has an accounting background, and his primary task since taking over as treasurer has been cash and short-term liability management. Thus, he is somewhat apprehensive about his new assignment, an apprehension that is heightened by the fact that one board member is a well-regarded University of Florida finance professor.

Clark began by reviewing Southern's 2009 financial statements, which are presented in Exhibit 16.1 in simplified form. Next, he assembled the following data:

1. Southern's long-term debt consists of 7.5 percent coupon, BBB-rated, semiannual payment bonds with 15 years remaining to maturity. The bonds recently traded at a price of $956.31 per $1,000 par value bond. The bonds are callable in five years at par value plus a call premium of one year's interest, for a total of $1,075.
2. The founders have an aversion to short-term debt, so the company uses such debt only to fund cyclical working capital needs. The company's financial plan calls for the issue of 30-year bonds to meet long-term debt needs.
3. Southern's federal-plus-state tax rate is 40 percent.
4. Southern's last dividend (D_o) was $0.18, and most analysts predict the company's dividend to grow at a relatively constant annual rate somewhere in the range

of 8 percent to 12 percent. Southern's common stock now sells at a price of $5.25 per share. The company has 10 million common shares outstanding.
5. Over the last few years, Southern has averaged a 20 percent return on equity and has paid out about 50 percent of its net income as dividends.
6. The current yield curve on U.S. Treasury securities is as follows:

Term to Maturity	Yield
3 months	2.5%
6 months	3.0
9 months	3.3
1 year	3.5
5 years	4.0
10 years	4.5
15 years	4.8
20 years	5.0
25 years	5.1
30 years	5.2

7. A prominent investment banking firm has recently estimated the expected rate of return on the S&P 500 Index to be 11 percent.
8. Southern's historical beta, as measured by several analysts who follow the stock, falls in the range of 1.3 to 1.5.
9. The required rate of return on an average (A-rated, beta = 1.0) company's long-term debt is 7 percent.
10. Southern's market value target capital structure calls for 35 percent long-term debt and 65 percent common stock.
11. Clark is aware of a third method (in addition to the capital asset pricing and discounted cash flow models) for estimating a firm's cost of equity: the bond yield plus risk-premium method. Here, a risk premium is added to the firm's own before-tax cost-of-debt estimate to obtain an estimate of the cost of equity. Note

Case 16: Southern Homecare 125

that the risk premium used here is not the market risk premium, which is applied to the risk-free rate. Rather, the risk premium reflects the difference between an average firm's cost of equity and its cost of debt.

12. About 60 percent of Southern's operating assets are used by the Healthcare Services Division, and 40 percent are used by the Information Systems Division. Management's best estimate of the beta of its Healthcare Services Division is 1.0.

Assume that Clark has hired you as a consultant to develop Southern's overall corporate cost of capital. You will have to meet with the financial VP and, possibly, with the president and the full board of directors (including the founders and the finance professor) to present your findings and answer any questions they might have.

In addition to the standard analysis, several issues related to the cost of capital estimate were raised at the last executive committee meeting. First, it is clear that cost of capital estimates are subject to significant uncertainty. Although a point (single) estimate is necessary, it would also be useful to get some idea of the corporate cost of capital's uncertainty by estimating its potential range of values.

Second, the divisional presidents expressed concern that a single cost of capital will be applied across the company, regardless of any divisional risk differences. Clark has asked you to be sure to address their concerns. Specifically, he wants you to develop divisional costs of capital in addition to the overall corporate cost of capital.

Third, the founders of Southern are very concerned about the threat posed by home health care businesses started by not-for-profit hospitals because they have both cost (in the sense that they do not pay dividends) and tax advantages. To help assess the threat, Clark has asked you to use the information developed for Southern, along with the not-for-profit hospital data contained in Exhibit 16.2, to estimate the cost of capital for an average not-for-profit hospital's home health care business.

Finally, one of Southern's directors has expressed concern over the difference between the company's target capital structure and the current structure as reported on the balance sheet. Clark wondered if this should be a matter of concern. (Hint: Think about book values versus market values. Which of these values is most appropriate for capital structure and cost of capital analysis?)

EXHIBIT 16.1
Southern Homecare:
2009 Financial Statement
Extracts
(millions of dollars)

Balance Sheet:

Cash and marketable securities	$ 2.5	Accounts payable	$ 1.1
Accounts receivable	5.9	Accruals	1.0
Inventory	1.3	Notes payable	0.2
Current assets	$ 9.7	Current liabilities	$ 2.3
Net fixed assets	32.9	Long-term debt	20.0
		Common stock	20.3
Total assets	$42.6	Total claims	$42.6

Income Statement:

Net revenues	$80.6
Cash expenses	71.8
Depreciation	2.8
Taxable income	$ 6.0
Taxes	2.4
Net income	$ 3.6
Dividends	1.8
Additions to retained earnings	$ 1.8

EXHIBIT 16.2
Selected Not-for-Profit
Hospital Data

Average Long-Term Capital Structure:
30 percent debt
70 percent equity (fund capital)

Average Cost of Debt:
Interest rate on A-rated tax-exempt bonds = 5.0%

RN TEMP SERVICES, INC.
CAPITAL STRUCTURE ANALYSIS

17

RN Temp Services, Inc., franchises "rent-a-nurse" businesses to independent operators throughout the United States. The concept of the business is the same as other temporary help services, such as Manpower and Kelly Temporary Services, except that RN Temp Services deals only with registered nurses. (For an example of a company similar to RN Temp Services, Inc., see www.interimhealthcare.com.)

The rationale behind RN Temp Services is as follows:

1. Many healthcare providers, especially hospitals, have difficulty hiring and retaining nurses, so there is almost always a demand for nursing professionals. Hospitals are the largest employer of registered nurses, employing almost 60 percent of the roughly 2.5 million working nurses. Traditionally, hospitals have been the dominant employer of nurses, but now nurses have opportunities that were not even dreamed of a generation ago. Registered nurses can work as nurse practitioners, nurse anesthetists, or critical care or neonatal specialists, all of which are in high demand today. In addition, registered nurses can work in home health agencies, nursing homes, utilization review positions, physicians' offices or outpatient surgery centers, and a multitude of other nonhospital settings such as schools. Of all the work settings, hospitals are

generally considered to be the least desirable because of the hard work, rigid work conditions, and irregular working hours. (For more information about the nursing profession, see the American Nurses Association website at www.nursingworld.org.)

2. Providers generally want to minimize fixed costs, so any staffing requirements that may not be permanent in nature are often filled by temporary workers. Also, when vacancies occur among permanent workers, providers often need temporary nurses to carry the load until the vacancies are filled with permanent personnel.

3. Although nursing salaries have increased over the past ten years, real wages have barely kept up with inflation. Furthermore, a large number of nurses have quit the profession for a variety of reasons, including family responsibilities. Many of these nurses are willing to work occasionally but not on a permanent basis. About one in five nurses works on a part-time basis.

4. Typically, the nurses who want to work on a selective basis have spouses who provide family coverage health insurance. Also, these nurses do not require extensive fringe benefits such as pension plans or paid vacations, and because they are part-time workers, they are not eligible for unemployment insurance or workers' compensation. Thus, if the average fringe-benefit package paid for permanent nurses is, say, 25 percent of salary, a temporary services company could offer a salary to its nurses 5 percent higher than can providers; could "rent" the nurses out at 5 percent less than it costs providers to hire permanent nurses, including all fringe benefits; and could pocket what remains of the 15 percent spread after administrative costs are paid. Note, however, that the actual rates charged by RN Temp Service's franchisees are related more to local supply-and-demand conditions than to costs.

Franchisees buy the exclusive right to use the RN Temp Services name within a specified territory from RN Temp Services, Inc., the franchisor. In addition, franchisees receive marketing and management support from RN Temp Services as well as the right to lease computers and other office equipment under relatively favorable terms. Finally, franchisees can purchase expendable office supplies directly from RN Temp Services, at substantial savings from retail prices.

To start operations, a franchisee recruits a pool of nurses from the local labor market. Then, when a client needs a temporary nurse, the local manager matches the client's specific needs with a qualified nurse from the pool. The bill for services is sent to the client by the franchisee based on the number of hours—verified by a timecard—that the nurse works for the client. The client has no responsibility for the nurse's salary or fringe benefits; this is all handled by the RN Temp Services franchisee.

Tiffany Radcliff, a registered nurse from Albuquerque who left the profession to get an MBA from the University of New Mexico, founded RN Temp Services in 1990. The firm grew rapidly from its base in Albuquerque, first by expanding operations into different cities across the Southwest and then by franchising into other parts of the country. Tiffany was a devout believer in the virtues of equity financing. Although the firm had issued debt periodically, especially to finance company-owned business expansion, Tiffany always used the firm's free cash flow to retire the debt as soon as possible. Recent growth has involved franchising, in which the franchisee puts up the required capital, and hence outside capital has not been needed for several years.

Tiffany believes that her firm's high-growth days are over. First, numerous companies that offer competing services have appeared on the scene. Second, the number of hospitals, which are her primary clients, has declined over the years since she founded the firm, and a meaningful increase in hospital beds is unlikely in the foreseeable future. Third, many hospitals have created "flexible staffing pools" for nurses, which, for all practical purposes, are in-house temporary work agencies. Finally, many large employers of nurses are recruiting internationally, which lessens the demand for temporary workers. Thus, Tiffany expects the firm's earnings to grow relatively slowly in the future.

RN Temp Services has 10 million shares of common stock outstanding, which are traded in the over-the-counter market. The current share price is $1.20, so the total market value of the firm's equity is $12 million. The book value of equity is also $12 million, so the stock now sells at its book value. The firm's federal-plus-state tax rate is 40 percent. Tiffany owns 20 percent of the outstanding stock, and others in the management group own an additional 10 percent.

Tiffany's financial manager, Paul Duncan, has been preaching for years that RN Temp Services should use some debt in its capital structure. "After all," says Paul, "everybody else uses debt, and some of our competitors use over 50 percent debt financing. Also, an underleveraged company is exposed to a hostile takeover because raiders can use the firm's excess debt capacity to finance the bid."

If the firm were to recapitalize, the borrowed funds would be used to repurchase stock in the open market, as the funds are not needed to grow the business. Tiffany's reaction to Paul's prodding is cautious, but she is willing to give Paul the chance to prove his point. Paul has worked with Tiffany for the past six years and knows that the only way he can convince her that the firm should use debt financing is to conduct a comprehensive capital structure analysis.

To begin, Paul arranged for a joint meeting with an investment banker who specializes in corporate financing for service companies. After several hours, the pair agreed on the estimates for the relationships between the use of debt financing and RN Temp Services's capital costs, which are shown in Exhibit 17.1. Additionally, Paul obtained industry capitalization data for companies that franchise professional services along with the matching debt ratings on the basis of rough guidance given by S&P Ratings Services. These data are contained in Exhibit 17.2.

Although RN Temp Services' earnings before interest and taxes (EBIT) is expected to be $3 million in 2010, there is some uncertainty in the estimate, as indicated by the following probability distribution:

Probability	EBIT
0.25	$2,500,000
0.50	3,000,000
0.25	3,500,000

On the basis of previous conversations, Paul knows that Tiffany has two major concerns regarding the use of debt financing. First, she is concerned about the impact of debt financing on the firm's reported profitability—that is, the impact of debt financing on net income and return on equity as reported in the firm's financial statements. Furthermore, any risk implications to stockholders must be identified. To help in this regard, Paul plans to construct partial income statements (beginning with EBIT) for four levels of debt as measured by the book value Total debt/Total assets ratio: zero, 25 percent, 50 percent, and 75 percent. For this analysis, which will not be used to make the actual capital structure decision, Paul intends to use a cost of debt of 10 percent regardless of the amount of debt financing used.

In addition to financial statement effects, Tiffany is obviously concerned about the potential impact of debt financing on the firm's stock price. To help address this issue, Paul is aware of a technique that can be used to value zero-growth firms at different debt levels. Clearly, the results of this analysis do not apply exactly to RN Temp Services, which is expected to experience slow growth, as opposed to zero growth, over the coming years. Here are the equations used in the analysis:

$$E = [EBIT - (R(R_d) \times D)](1 - T)/R(R_e). \quad (1)$$
$$V = E + D. \quad (2)$$
$$P = (V - D_0)/n_0. \quad (3)$$
$$n_1 = n_0 - D/P. \quad (4)$$

In these equations,

- E = market value of equity
- $EBIT$ = earnings before interest and taxes
- $R(R_d)$ = cost of debt
- D = market (and book) value of new debt
- D_0 = market value of old debt
- T = tax rate
- $R(R_e)$ = cost of equity
- V = total market value
- P = stock price after recapitalization
- n_0 = number of shares before recapitalization
- n_1 = number of shares after recapitalization

Paul is also concerned about potential changes in the healthcare industry and how they might affect the basic business risk of RN Temp Services should they occur. Exhibit 17.3 contains leverage/cost estimates at alternative business-risk levels. Note that the values in Exhibit

17.3 are for what-if analysis purposes only. The best current estimates of the financing costs at alternative debt levels are given in Exhibit 17.1.

Finally, because the capital structure decision is heavily influenced by a host of qualitative factors as well as the actions of other businesses in the industry, Paul uncovered the following additional industry data:

1. The average healthcare franchise business has a times-interest-earned (TIE) ratio of 4.0.
2. RN Temp Services, Inc., has a current cash and marketable securities balance of $500,000. The average healthcare franchise business has cash and marketable securities on hand that is equal to 70 percent of its annual interest payment.

Put yourself in Paul's shoes and see if you can convince Tiffany that the business should use debt financing. Be sure to recommend the optimal amount for the firm and do not forget (1) that the no-growth model can be used only as a rough guide and (2) that subjective factors are as important as numerical analyses to the final decision.

Optional information: (Address this issue only if you are familiar with the following capital structure models.) Paul knows that Tiffany is familiar with capital structure theory and will want to know the value of the firm according to the Modigliani-Miller with corporate taxes model and the Miller model. Because most of the other board members are not familiar with capital structure decisions, conducting a tutorial on the issues involved will be necessary, including the difference between business and financial risk, the relationship between capital structure and earnings per share, and the additional qualitative factors that influence the decision. To ease comparisons, assume that the value of RN Temp Services, with zero debt financing, is $12 million in both models. Also, assume that the personal tax rates are 15 percent on stock income and 30 percent on debt income.

EXHIBIT 17.1
RN Temp Services, Inc.: Relationships Between the Level of Debt Financing and Capital Costs

Amount Borrowed	Cost of Debt	Cost of Equity
$ 0	—	15.0%
2,500,000	10.0%	15.5
5,000,000	11.0	16.5
7,500,000	13.0	18.0
10,000,000	16.0	20.0
12,500,000	20.0	25.0

EXHIBIT 17.2
Industry Average Data and Matching Debt Ratings

Percentile	Market Value Debt Ratio	Debt Rating
10th	10%	AAA
25th	25	AA
40th	35	A
Median	50	BBB
60th	65	BB
75th	75	B
90th	82	C

Note: The debt ratio is defined as Total debt/Total assets.

EXHIBIT 17.3
Level of Debt and Cost Estimates at Different Business-Risk Levels

Significant Increase in Business Risk:

Amount Borrowed	Cost of Debt	Cost of Equity
$ 0	—	16.0%
2,500,000	11.0%	17.0
5,000,000	13.0	19.0
7,500,000	16.0	22.0
10,000,000	20.0	26.0
12,500,000	25.0	31.0

Significant Decrease in Business Risk:

Amount Borrowed	Cost of Debt	Cost of Equity
$ 0	—	14.0%
2,500,000	9.0%	14.3
5,000,000	9.5	15.0
7,500,000	10.5	16.0
10,000,000	12.5	17.5
12,500,000	15.5	20.0

PORTLAND CANCER CENTER
LEASING DECISIONS

18

PORTLAND CANCER CENTER (the Center) is a nationally known not-for-profit inpatient and outpatient facility dedicated to the prevention and treatment of cancer. Specific treatment services include surgery, chemotherapy, bone marrow transplantation, radiation therapy, and photodynamic therapy.

For the past ten years, the Center has been working diligently to perfect noninvasive brain surgery techniques. One technique, Gamma Knife radiosurgery, was developed in the 1950s and 1960s by Dr. Lars Leksell, a prominent Swedish neurosurgeon. The first patient treatment site was opened in 1968 in Stockholm, while the first site in the United States was established in 1977 in Pittsburgh.

The Gamma Knife uses 201 separate radiation sources to treat certain brain cancers. Each of the radiation beams is quite weak and hence does not damage normal brain tissue, but when the separate beams are focused on a single point by a collimator helmet, the Gamma Knife delivers a dosage sufficient to be highly effective. The Gamma Knife is especially useful in the treatment of arteriovenous malformations, but it can also be used to treat certain types of benign tumors and even some small malignant lesions. The primary clinical benefit of the Gamma Knife is the significant reduction in the risk associated with traditional surgical procedures, in which the morbidity and mortality rate is substantial, especially for patients with deep lesions. In addition to treating cancer, the Gamma Knife can be used to treat functional disorders such as Parkinson's disease tremors and the pain that results from trigeminal neuralgia. (For more information about the Gamma Knife, including an informative video on Gamma Knife surgery, see the manufacturer's website at www.gammaknife.org.)

The procedure calls for a team approach, including a neurosurgeon, radiation physicist, radiologist, and radiation therapist. The neurosurgeon selects the patients appropriate for the procedure and performs the stereotactic process required to localize the target area. The radiation physicist works with a computer program to compute the appropriate dosimetry, while the radiologist performs a CT scan, MRI scan, angiogram, or a combination of the three to help the neurosurgeon localize the lesion.

The dosimetry calculations are especially complex. Because differing thicknesses of skull and brain will attenuate the beams in varying amounts, the amount of radiation applied is highly dependent on where the lesion is located and the size and shape of the patient's skull. The actual application of the radiation generally takes between 20 minutes and 2 hours, and the patient is generally released after only a short period of observation.

The Center plans to acquire a new Gamma Knife to replace its current model. The equipment has an invoice price of $3 million, including delivery and installation charges, and it falls into the modified accelerated cost recovery system (MACRS) five-year class, with current allowances of 0.20, 0.32, 0.19, 0.12, 0.11, and 0.06 in Years 1–6, respectively. The manufacturer of the equipment will provide a maintenance contract for $100,000 per year, payable at the beginning of each year, if the Center buys the equipment. Furthermore, the purchase could be financed by a four-year simple-interest conventional (taxable) bank note that carries an interest rate of 8 percent.

Regardless of whether the equipment is purchased or leased, the Center's managers do not think that it will be used for more than four years, at which time the Center plans to open a new radiation therapy facility. Land on which to construct a larger facility has already been acquired, and the building should be ready for occupancy at that time. The new facility is designed to enable the Center to use several new radiosurgery procedures. Thus, the Gamma Knife replacement is viewed as a "bridge," to serve only until the new facility is ready four years from now. The expected physical life of the equipment is ten years, but medical equipment of this nature is subject to unpredictable technological obsolescence.

After considerable debate among the Center's managers, they concluded that there is a 25 percent probability that the residual (salvage) value after four years will be $500,000; a 50 percent probability that it will be $1 million; and a 25 percent probability that it will be $2 million, which makes the residual value quite risky. Because the residual value is judged to have high risk, a 5 percentage point risk adjustment will be added to the base discount rate used on the other lease-analysis flows to obtain the appropriate rate for the residual value flows.

GB Financing (GBF), a leasing company that is partially owned by the manufacturer, has presented an initial offer to the Center to lease the equipment for annual payments of $675,000, with the first payment due on delivery and installation and additional payments due at the beginning of each succeeding year of the four-year lease term. This rental price includes a service contract under which the equipment will be maintained in good working order. GBF will buy the equipment from the manufacturer under the same terms that were offered to the Center, and GBF will have to enter into a maintenance contract with the manufacturer for $100,000 per year. (For more information on leasing healthcare equipment, see the GE financing website at www.gehealthcarefinance.com.)

Unlike the Center, GBF forecasts a $1.5 million residual value. Its estimate is based on the following facts: (1) No technology currently exists that will make the Gamma Knife obsolete; (2) the equipment has a physical life estimated to be two and one-half times longer than the four-year lease term; and (3) GBF is more skilled than the Center in selling used equipment, especially Gamma Knives. GBF's federal-plus-state tax rate is 40 percent, and if the lease is not written, GBF could invest the funds in a four-year term loan of similar risk that yields 8 percent before taxes.

Randall Williams, the Center's chief financial officer, has the final say on all of the business's lease-versus-purchase decisions, but the actual analysis of the relevant data will be conducted by the Center's capital funds manager, Vanessa Seagle. In the past, Randall and Vanessa have more or less agreed on analytical methodologies, but in discussing this lease analysis, they ended up in a heated discussion about the appropriate discount rate to use in the analysis.

Randall argued that the cash flows associated with performing stereotactic radiosurgery are uncertain. He is convinced that payers are not going to be nearly as generous in the future as they have been in the past in funding such procedures, so the revenue stream is highly speculative. Accordingly, he thinks that a high discount rate should be used in the analysis. Vanessa, on the other hand, believes that leasing is a substitute for other financing, which means a blend of debt and equity capital. Consequently, she believes that the lease-analysis cash flows should be discounted at the Center's corporate cost of capital, 10 percent. However, both Randall and Vanessa are possibly wrong. In addition to the discount rate dispute, there is also some disagreement about how the lease would be handled on the Center's financial statements, so that has to be resolved.

Both Randall and Vanessa think that lessees should not blindly accept the first offer made by potential lessors but should conduct a complete analysis from the viewpoint of both parties and then, using this knowledge, negotiate the best deal possible. Thus, knowing the range of lease payments that is acceptable to both parties is important.

There is a possibility that the Center will move to its new radiation facility earlier than anticipated and hence prior to the expiration of the lease. Furthermore, if the neurosurgeon who is the primary user of this procedure leaves the staff and is not immediately replaced, the equipment will be useless. Thus, Randall is considering asking GBF to include a cancellation clause in the lease contract. Under such a clause, the Center will be able to return the equipment to GBF at any time during the lease term after giving a minimum 30-day notice. Before negotiations begin, the Center must assess the impact of such a clause on the riskiness of the lease to both parties and any consequences it might have on the terms of the lease.

In addition to a cancellation clause, Randall is aware that many lessors are now writing per-procedure leases, in which the lease payment is tied to the number of procedures performed rather than a fixed amount. Randall wonders what the consequences would be for both the lessee and lessor if this type of lease were used instead of a conventional lease. GBF has quoted a per-procedure lease rate of $7,000 based on an expected annual volume of 100 procedures. However, past experience indicated that volume could easily be as low as 70 or as high as 130 procedures. Based on current charges and reimbursement rates, the Center expects to realize net revenue per procedure of roughly $10,000.

There also has been some discussion about obtaining tax-exempt financing for the Gamma Knife should it be purchased. If so, the cost of tax-exempt (municipal) debt would be only 5 percent. To complicate matters even more, the Center currently has more than $5 million in excess funds invested in marketable securities that earn 3 percent, and these funds, rather than debt financing, could be used to purchase the equipment.

Finally, Randall's brother-in-law, who works at GBF, found out that GBF will probably obtain a $1.5 million simple-interest loan, which GBF will use to leverage the lease. The terms of this loan have not been finalized, but the bank has indicated that the interest rate would be in the range of 7–9 percent. Such leveraging could affect the Center's ability to negotiate lower lease payments, so understanding the impact of leveraging from the perspectives of both the lessee and the lessor is important.

Assume that you have been hired as a consultant to recommend a course of action for the Gamma Knife acquisition. Prepare a report that addresses all of the issues raised by the parties involved and makes a final recommendation regarding the acquisition.

*Capital
Investment*

PALMS HOSPITAL

19

TRADITIONAL PROJECT ANALYSIS

PALMS HOSPITAL is a 250-bed, investor-owned hospital located in Islamorada, Florida, which is known as the "The Sport Fishing Capital of the World." The hospital was founded in 1946 by Rob Winslow, a prominent Florida physician, on his return from service in World War II. Dr. Winslow relinquished control of the hospital in 1967 while it was still small and in a relatively quiet setting. However, in recent years, the Florida Keys have experienced a population explosion, which has fostered high economic growth as well as a continuing need for more healthcare services. Today, under a succession of excellent chief executive officers, the hospital is acknowledged to be one of the leading healthcare providers in the area.

The hospital's management is currently evaluating a proposed ambulatory (outpatient) surgery center. (For more information on ambulatory surgery, see the Ambulatory Surgery Center Association website at www.ascassociation.org). More than 80 percent of all outpatient surgery is performed by specialists in gastroenterology, gynecology, ophthalmology, otolaryngology, orthopedics, plastic surgery, and urology. Ambulatory surgery requires an average of about one and one-half hours: Minor procedures take about one hour or less, and major procedures take about two or more hours. About 60 percent of the procedures are performed under general anesthesia, 30 percent under local anesthesia, and 10 percent under regional or spinal anesthesia. In general, operating rooms are built in pairs so that a patient can be prepped in one room while the surgeon is completing a procedure in the other room.

The outpatient surgery market has experienced significant growth since the first ambulatory surgery center opened in 1970. By 1990, about 2.5 million procedures were being performed at stand-alone outpatient centers, but by 2009 the number had grown to more than 20 million. This growth has been fueled primarily by three factors. First, rapid advancements in technology have enabled many procedures that were historically performed in inpatient surgical suites to be switched to outpatient settings. This shift was caused mainly by advances in laser, laparoscopic, endoscopic, and arthroscopic technologies. Second, Medicare has been aggressive in approving new minimally invasive surgery techniques, so the number of Medicare patients who use outpatient surgery services has grown substantially. Finally, patients prefer outpatient surgeries because they are more convenient, and third-party payers prefer them because they are less costly.

All of these factors have led to a situation in which the number of inpatient surgeries has remained more or less flat over the last 20 years, while the number of outpatient procedures has continuously grown at more than 10 percent annually. Rapid growth in the number of outpatient surgeries has been accompanied by a corresponding growth in the number of outpatient facilities nationwide. The number currently stands at about 5,000, so competition in many areas has become intense. Somewhat surprisingly, no outpatient surgery center exists in the hospital's immediate service area, although the rumor is that local surgeons are exploring the feasibility of a physician-owned facility.

Palms Hospital currently owns a parcel of land adjacent to its facility that is a perfect location for the surgery center. The hospital bought the land five years ago for $150,000, and last year the hospital spent (and expensed for tax purposes) $25,000 to clear the land and put in sewer and utility lines. If sold in today's market, the land will bring in $200,000, net of all fees, commissions, and taxes. Land prices have been extremely volatile, so the hospital's standard procedure is to assume a salvage value equal to the current value of the land. Of course, land is not depreciated for either book or tax purposes.

The surgery center building, which will house four operating suites, costs $5 million and the equipment costs an additional $5 million, for a total of $10 million. For ease, assume that both the building and the equipment fall into the modified accelerated cost recovery system (MACRS) five-year class for tax-depreciation purposes. (In reality, the building has to be depreciated over a much longer period than the equipment.) The project will probably have a long life, but the hospital typically assumes a five-year life in its capital budgeting analyses and then approximates the value of the cash flows beyond Year 5 by including a terminal, or salvage, value in the analysis. To estimate the salvage value, the hospital typically uses the market value of the building and equipment after five years, which for this project is estimated to be $5 million before taxes, excluding the land value. (Note that taxes must be paid on the difference between an asset's salvage value and its tax book value at termination. For example, if an asset that costs $10,000 is depreciated to $5,000 and then sold for $7,000, the firm owes taxes on the $2,000 excess in salvage value over tax book value.)

The expected volume at the surgery center is 20 procedures a day. The average charge per procedure is expected to be $1,500, but charity care, bad debts, managed care plan discounts, and other allowances lower the net revenue amount to $1,000. The center will be open five days a week, 50 weeks a year, for a total of 250 days a year. As detailed in Exhibit 19.1, labor costs to run the surgery center are estimated at $918,000 per year, including fringe benefits. Utilities, including hazardous waste disposal, add another $50,000 in annual costs.

If the surgery center is built, the hospital's cash overhead costs will increase by $36,000 annually, primarily for housekeeping and buildings and grounds maintenance. In addition, the center will be allocated $25,000 of the hospital's current $2.8 million in administrative overhead costs. On average, each procedure will require $200 in expendable medical supplies, including anesthetics. Although the hospital's inventories and receivables will rise slightly if the center is constructed, its accruals and payables will also increase. The overall change in net working capital is expected to be small and hence not material to the analysis. The hospital's marginal federal-plus-state tax rate is 40 percent.

Inflation is one of the most difficult factors to deal with in project analysis. Both input costs and charges in the healthcare industry have been rising at about twice the rate of overall inflation. Furthermore, inflationary pressures have been highly variable. Because of the difficulties involved in forecasting inflation rates, the hospital begins each analysis by assuming that both revenues and costs, except for depreciation, will increase at a constant rate. Under current conditions, this rate is assumed to be 3 percent.

When the project was mentioned briefly at the last meeting of the hospital's board of directors, several questions were raised. In particular, one board member wanted to make sure that a complete risk analysis, including sensitivity and scenario analyses, is performed before the proposal is presented to the board. Recently, the board was forced to close a daycare center that appeared to be profitable when analyzed two years ago but turned out to be a big money loser. The board does not want a repeat of that occurrence. Another board member countered that she thought the hospital was putting too much faith in the numbers: "After all," she pointed out, "that is what got us into trouble on the daycare center. We need to start worrying more about how projects fit into our strategic vision and how they affect the services that we currently offer."

Another director, who is also the hospital's chief of medicine, expressed concern over the impact of the ambulatory surgery center on the current volume of inpatient surgeries. This concern prompted an analysis by the surgery department head, who reported that an outpatient surgery center could siphon off up to $1 million in cash revenues annually. When pressed, the department head estimated that such a reduction in volume could also lead to a $500,000 reduction in annual cash expenses.

To develop the data needed for the risk analysis, Jules Bergman, the hospital's director of capital budgeting, met with department heads of surgery, marketing, and facilities. After several sessions, they concluded that three input variables are highly uncertain: number of procedures per day, average revenue per procedure, and building/equipment salvage value. If another entity entered the local ambulatory surgery market, the number of procedures could be as low as 10 per day. Conversely, if acceptance is strong and no competing centers are built, the number of procedures could be as high as 25 per day, compared to the most likely value of 20 per day.

The average net revenue amount, with an expected value of $1,000, is a function of the types of procedures performed and the amount of managed care penetration. If surgery severity is high (i.e., if a higher number of complicated procedures than anticipated are performed) and managed care penetration remains low, then the average revenue could be as high as $1,200. Conversely, if the severity is lower than expected and managed care penetration increases, the average revenue could be as low as $800. Finally, if real estate and medical equipment values stay strong, the building/equipment salvage value could be as high as $6 million, but if the market weakens, the salvage value could be as low as $4 million, compared to an expected value of $5 million.

Jules also discussed the probabilities of the various scenarios with the medical and marketing staffs, but after considerable debate no consensus could be reached. To add to the confusion, one member of the medical staff, who had just returned from a University of Michigan executive program on financial management, questioned why the scenario analysis had to be confined to just three scenarios. "Why not five or seven?" he queried. Additionally, he said that the executive program had taught him a good way to assess the impact of inflation on project profitability, which is to create and analyze an inflation impact table, such as the one shown in Exhibit 19.2.

To help with the risk-incorporation phase of the analysis, Jules consulted with Mark Hauser, the hospital's chief financial officer, about both the risk inherent in the hospital's average project and how the hospital typically adjusts for risk. Mark told Jules that based on historical scenario analysis data that use worst, most likely, and best case values, the hospital's average project has a coefficient of variation of net present value (NPV) in the range of 1.0–2.0 and that the hospital typically adds or subtracts 4 percentage points to its 10 percent corporate cost of capital to adjust for differential project risk.

Assume that Palms Hospital has hired you as a financial consultant. Your task is to conduct a complete project analysis on the ambulatory surgery center and then present your findings and recommendations to the hospital's board of directors.

Optional: This case is well suited for the application of Monte Carlo simulation. If you are familiar with this risk-assessment technique and have access to the appropriate add-in software, apply it to this case. (Note that Palisade Corporation, the maker of @RISK, offers a free demonstration version of this popular Monte Carlo simulation add-in. See www.palisade.com.)

EXHIBIT 19.1
Palms Hospital: Projected Surgery Center Staffing Requirements

Position	Annual Salary	FTEs	Total Salary
Executive director	$60,000	1	$ 60,000
Director of nursing	50,000	1	50,000
Accounting clerk	35,000	1	35,000
Collections clerk	30,000	1	30,000
Scheduling clerk	25,000	1	25,000
Registered nurses	60,000	8	480,000
Nursing assistants	30,000	2	60,000
Transcriptionist	25,000	1	25,000
Total			$765,000
Plus 20 percent fringe benefit allowance			153,000
Total salaries and benefits			$918,000

FTE: full-time equivalent

EXHIBIT 19.2
Inflation Impact Table

		\multicolumn{5}{c}{Level of Revenue Inflation}
		0%	3.0%	6.0%	9.0%	12.0%
Level of Cost Inflation	0%	NPV	NPV	NPV	NPV	NPV
	3.0	NPV	NPV	NPV	NPV	NPV
	6.0	NPV	NPV	NPV	NPV	NPV
	9.0	NPV	NPV	NPV	NPV	NPV
	12.0	NPV	NPV	NPV	NPV	NPV

NPV: net present value

AMERICAN REHABILITATION CENTERS

STAGED ENTRY ANALYSIS

20

AMERICAN REHABILITATION CENTERS (ARC) is one of the nation's leading providers of outpatient rehabilitative medicine. It was founded in 1984 in Phoenix, Arizona, by a group of five individuals who recognized the need for cost-effective alternatives to traditional hospital-based rehabilitative services. This vision has become the hallmark for the company, and it continues today to provide the highest-quality, most cost-effective care available. (For more information on rehabilitative medicine, see the American Academy of Physical Medicine and Rehabilitation website at www.aapmr.org.)

In its quest to lower the costs of rehabilitative services, ARC uses the latest in noninvasive treatment procedures, which reduces direct costs and results in quicker recoveries. In addition, the company encourages patients to begin aggressive rehabilitation as early as possible, which helps them return to normal functioning more quickly than under conventional treatment protocols. In spite of ARC's relatively short history, its strategy has worked wonders, and ARC quickly expanded from a local to a regional to a national company. Today, ARC is a multibillion-dollar, publicly traded company with nearly 750 locations in all 50 states, Puerto Rico, the United Kingdom, and Australia.

For several years, ARC's board of directors has been considering expanding its service line to include sports medicine. The American College of Sports Medicine defines sports medicine as the physiological, biomechanical, psychological, and pathological phenomena associated with exercise and sports. (For more information on sports medicine, see the American College of Sports Medicine website at www.acsm.org.) Because a considerable degree of commonality exists between rehabilitative and sports medicine services, expansion into this rapidly growing area of healthcare seemed natural.

ARC's board is examining two proposals related to the expansion. Proposal A involves a single, large investment that will immediately give the company a national presence in sports medicine. In essence, all of the current rehabilitation facilities deemed suitable to offer sports medicine services will be renovated, equipped, and staffed, as required, to offer sports medicine services. The amount of capital investment at each of the company's earmarked locations will vary significantly, but the average cost is estimated at about $800,000 per facility. With roughly 500 locations identified as suitable for the sports medicine business line, the estimated cost of Proposal A is in the vicinity of $400 million. Although the profitability analysis of Proposal A is only preliminary, its internal rate of return is thought to be in the range of 20–25 percent.

Proposal B, on the other hand, involves a more deliberate, two-stage approach to the expansion. Stage 1 of Proposal B calls for a trial program in which only one of ARC's nine regions will offer sports medicine services. If the results of Stage 1 meet the company's expectations, Stage 2, which calls for the expansion of sports medicine services into the remaining eight regions, will be implemented.

Proposal A requires a much larger capital investment than does Stage 1 of Proposal B. However, Proposal B is more costly than Proposal A overall, even when time value is considered, because Proposal A's large up-front investment leads to greater efficiencies in contracting, construction, recruitment, and marketing. In spite of Proposal A's cost advantage, several board members are concerned about the wisdom of Proposal A because it requires ARC to make a large investment in a business line that is new to the company. Other board members, however, see no difference between rehabilitation and sports medicine services, prompting a board member to say, "Healthcare is healthcare."

The primary task at hand is to evaluate Proposal B, which includes the trial program and possible expansion into all service regions. To date, ARC has spent $7 million to develop a sports medicine service concept that matches its approach to rehabilitative medicine. Of the

$7 million, $2 million have been expensed for tax purposes, while the remaining $5 million have been capitalized and will be amortized over the five-year operating life of Stage 1. According to a specific IRS ruling requested by ARC, if neither Proposal A nor B is implemented, the $5 million could be immediately expensed.

If it decides to go ahead with Stage 1, ARC will immediately spend $2 million to perform local labor-market studies to ensure that the locations identified for the sports medicine program could be staffed. The next step is to buy the land needed at locations where totally new facilities are required. In total, land acquisition costs, which are assumed to occur at the end of Year 1, are expected to be $10 million. New construction and renovations at the chosen locations will take place during Years 2 and 3, and equipment will be installed during the last quarter of Year 3. Also, additional personnel, as needed, will be hired at the end of Year 3. The total amount needed for new buildings, renovations to existing buildings, and equipment (plus a relatively small amount for recruitment) is estimated to be $50 million. For planning purposes, half of this amount is assumed to be spent at the end of Year 2 and the other half at the end of Year 3.

Although any new building falls into the modified accelerated cost recovery system (MACRS) 39-year class, for simplicity both the buildings and equipment needed are assumed to fall into the MACRS seven-year class. Appropriate depreciation allowances are given in Exhibit 20.1. ARC will begin to depreciate the buildings and equipment during Year 4, the year in which the trial sports medicine program will be initiated. The trial program will be evaluated at the beginning of Year 6. If the results are satisfactory, the program will be expanded to the remaining eight regions. If the program does not meet expectations, it will be terminated at the end of Year 8. If terminated, the land will have an estimated market value of $10 million at the end of Year 8, while the buildings and equipment will have a market value of $30 million.

ARC's marketing department has projected two demand scenarios for Stage 1. If demand for the sports medicine program is poor, total revenues are forecasted to be $40 million for Year 4, the first year of operations. However, if demand is good, revenues are expected to be $60 million. At this point, the best guess is that there is a 50 percent chance of poor demand and a 50 percent chance of good demand. If demand is good, revenues are expected to increase by 6 percent each year after Year 4. If demand is poor, revenue growth is expected to be only 3 percent.

In terms of operating costs, variable costs are expected to be 30 percent of revenues. Fixed costs (other than depreciation), which are expected to total $25 million in Year 4, are forecasted to increase after the initial year of operations at the anticipated overall rate of inflation, 2 percent.

If the board approves Stage 2, ARC will spend an additional $480 million on land, buildings, and equipment to expand into the other eight regions. This expenditure will be evenly split between Years 6 and 7. As shown below, the net cash inflows forecasted for Stage 2 depend on the demand scenario:

End of Year	Net Cash Flow		
	High Demand	Medium Demand	Low Demand
6	($240,000,000)	($240,000,000)	($240,000,000)
7	(240,000,000)	(240,000,000)	(240,000,000)
8	210,000,000	160,000,000	70,000,000
9	228,000,000	170,000,000	75,000,000
10	241,000,000	175,000,000	75,000,000
11	256,000,000	180,000,000	75,000,000
12	500,000,000	350,000,000	150,000,000

Note that the net cash flows have been "bumped up" in Year 9 to reflect the cash flows from those facilities in the test region. Also, note that the project is expected to last beyond Year 12, and an allowance for the value of these future cash flows is embedded in the Year 12 cash flows.

The estimated probabilities of the Stage 2 demand scenarios are related to the response to the Stage 1 trial program. If acceptance is poor in Stage 1, there is a 10 percent probability that demand will be high during Stage 2, a 30 percent probability that demand will be medium, and a 60 percent probability that demand will be low. However, if acceptance during Stage 1 is good, there is a 60 percent probability that demand will be high during Stage 2, a 30 percent probability that demand will be medium, and a 10 percent probability that demand will be low. Of course, these expectations may change over time as new information becomes available. Furthermore, the actual demand scenario for Stage 2 is not expected to be known until midway through Year 8, after the program has been in operation nationally for six months.

ARC's current income tax rate is 40 percent, and this rate is projected to remain roughly constant into the future. The firm's corporate cost of capital is 10.0 percent, but ARC adjusts this amount up or down by 3 percentage points to adjust for project risk. ARC defines low-risk projects as those that have a coefficient of variation (CV) of net present value less than 0.5, average-risk projects have CVs in the range of 0.5–1.5, and high-risk projects have CVs more than 1.5.

One of the most important advantages of staged entry is that new information will become available throughout the investment period. ARC's managers recognize this feature and believe that they will have a better estimate of the Stage 2 probabilities and cash flows before making the Year 6 investment. Even if Stage 2 is undertaken, there is some possibility that the project could be abandoned at the end of Year 8 if the low demand scenario materializes. If the project is abandoned at that point, the best estimate for the Year 8 cash flow is $420 million. The uncertainty of whether or not abandonment will occur lies more in the politics than in the economics of the decision. In the past, ARC's managers were not so inclined to admit mistakes and cut losses, so some doubt lingers about whether the abandonment decision will be made even if it is the financially right thing to do at the time.

Assume that you have been hired as a consultant to analyze the situation regarding the sports medicine program and then make a recommendation to ARC's board of directors regarding the best course of action. In addition to a detailed analysis of Proposal B, you have been asked to compare the relative merits of Proposals A and B.

EXHIBIT 20.1 MACRS Depreciation Rates

MACRS Class	Recovery Year				
	1	2	3	4	5
7-year	14.3%	24.5%	17.5%	12.5%	8.9%

Note: For ease, these allowances were rounded to the nearest one-tenth of 1 percent. In actual applications, the allowances would not be rounded.

COOK COUNTY HEALTH SYSTEM

MAKE OR BUY ANALYSIS

21

COOK COUNTY HEALTH SYSTEM (the System) is a large not-for-profit healthcare holding company that operates both not-for-profit and for-profit subsidiaries in Chicago and its surrounding area. The not-for-profit subsidiaries consist of four acute care hospitals (Metropolitan Memorial, Des Plaines General, Winnetka Memorial, and Skokie General) and one service company (SUPPORT). SUPPORT provides various services, such as food, laundry, and medical waste disposal, to the four hospitals. The single for-profit subsidiary, PROPERTIES, operates several for-profit businesses, but its primary business line is real estate development, particularly medical office buildings.

The System's chief executive officer, Susan Richards, has been thinking about the company's printing situation for some time. The System has a print shop, which currently operates under SUPPORT, that provides some of the printing required by the hospitals, but it does not have the capabilities to do all the work required. As shown in Exhibit 21.1, the System currently (2009) spends about $830,000 a year on commercial contract printing, some of which could be done in-house if the System expanded its printing capability.

Of the $830,000, about $132,000 represents graphics printing—annual reports, brochures, and other promotional material. Most of the graphics printing (about $119,000) could be moved in-house, but about 10 percent of the work (for example, the four-color annual report) will have to continue to be done by outside vendors.

Conversely, only about 30 percent of the almost $700,000 in forms printing, or about $209,000, could be moved in-house. The reason for this is that most forms printing requires specialized equipment and printing forms in-house is just not cost effective for businesses, except for very large companies. The System's print contracts (both graphics and forms) with vendors increased in dollar volume by about 5 percent (2 percent volume increase and 3 percent price increase) from 2008 to 2009, and this trend is expected to continue into the foreseeable future.

In 2009, the in-house print shop handled $42,837 in hospital billings. (To avoid any potential problems with SUPPORT's not-for-profit status, the print shop currently performs work exclusively for the System's four not-for-profit hospitals.) The print shop bills for materials only, but because material costs represent, on average, 30 percent of commercial vendors' total billings, the print shop currently does about $42,837/0.30 = $142,790 in annual work on a commercial billing basis. The equipment in the print shop has a current market value of $400,000, and the print shop generates about $40,000 in annual depreciation expense for tax purposes.

To move 90 percent of the vendor graphics printing and 30 percent of the vendor forms printing in-house, the System will have to invest in additional printing equipment. The capital investment necessary for expansion can vary significantly depending on whether new or used equipment is purchased, the type of main press selected, and whether only essential or nice-to-have equipment is purchased. Exhibit 21.2 summarizes the equipment capital-investment requirements. Note that the old equipment will be retained if the print shop is expanded. Also, the new equipment will generate tax depreciation of about $25,000 per year, and the required delivery van will cost $2,000 a year to operate (in 2009 dollars).

The print shop is currently located in a leased space adjacent to Metropolitan Memorial, the largest of the four hospitals. The cost of this site is $10 per square foot per year. The print shop occupies 2,000 square feet, and hence current building costs are $20,000 in annual lease payments plus an additional $200 monthly in utilities and insurance. Unfortunately, this site cannot be expanded, and hence new space is required if the print shop is to increase its capacity. Suitable space in a good location can be leased at the same rental rate ($10 per square foot per year), but the new print shop will require 3,500 square feet, increasing the annual lease cost by $35,000 − $20,000 = $15,000. (Assume that lease payments occur at the beginning of each year.)

In addition, the new space will require $30,000 in initial remodeling costs and an additional $100 per month in utilities and insurance costs (in 2009 dollars). Note that all leases are negotiated for a five-year period, so lease payments are not affected by inflation, which is expected to average about 3 percent per year.

The expanded print shop will require an increase in labor costs of $98,400; these costs are summarized in Exhibit 21.3. Labor costs to run the current print shop amount to $50,000 annually, and all current print shop personnel will be retained if the expansion takes place.

After discussing the print shop situation with her chief financial officer, Susan defined three possible print shop alternatives:

1. Close the print shop completely, and use outside vendors for all printing.
2. Expand the print shop as envisioned. Essentially, this means expanding the print shop and performing all feasible work in-house. Under this proposal, the print shop will remain under SUPPORT, the System's not-for-profit service subsidiary. Thus, there would be no tax consequences.
3. Expand the print shop as in Alternative 2. However, all printing activities will be transferred to PROPERTIES, the System's for-profit subsidiary. In this situation, capital expenses, such as depreciation and lease payments, will be tax deductible. The primary motivation behind this alternative is to permit the print shop to enter the for-profit commercial printing business.

Regarding Proposal 1, many outsiders to the hospital industry may be surprised at the amount of outsourcing that takes place. The business of running a hospital is extremely complicated, and many facets of its operations can be more efficiently run by companies that specialize in those areas. The three most common functions that are outsourced (by number of hospitals) are laundry, housekeeping, and food services. However, the list goes on and on. In fact, some hospitals are outsourcing to such a degree that they have created the position of COO — not chief operating officer but chief outsourcing officer.

The System's corporate cost of capital, which is dominated by hospital operations, is estimated to be 8 percent. However, the company also computes divisional costs of capital for each subsidiary. SUPPORT, the not-for-profit service subsidiary, has access to municipal debt that currently costs about 5.5 percent. Its target capital structure consists of 60 percent debt and 40 percent equity (fund) financing. Because SUPPORT has a captive business relationship with the System's four hospitals, it has relatively low business risk. Consequently, it has a relatively low cost of equity, 13 percent.

PROPERTIES, the for-profit subsidiary, cannot issue municipal debt. The bulk of its debt consists of mortgage loans provided by banks and insurance companies. Mortgage debt, which is secured by pledged property, has a relatively low interest rate for taxable debt. Currently, this rate is 7.5 percent. The subsidiary's combined federal-plus-state tax rate is 40 percent. Because PROPERTIES competes with other property development companies, its inherent business risk is high, and hence it has a relatively high cost of equity, 17 percent. However, its ability to use property as collateral for its debt financing gives it a relatively high debt capacity—about 75 percent. The System's capital budgeting policy guidelines call for all cash-flow analyses to be restricted to a five-year horizon with zero end-of-project salvage values. The rationale is that estimating cash flows any further into the future is just too difficult.

It is now December 2009, and the print shop analysis is due in one week. Thus, for ease, assume that all capital investment cash flows, as well as lease payments for 2010, occur at the beginning of 2010 (the end of 2009). Then, the five years of operating flows occur from 2010 through 2014. Also, the System's capital budgeting policy is to assume that all costs and prices that are not fixed by contract will increase at a 3 percent inflation rate. Thus, any 2009 dollar costs must be increased by 3 percent annually beginning in 2010. Furthermore, any 2009 volume amounts must be increased by 2 percent annually beginning in 2010.

In regard to the feasibility of entering the commercial printing business should the print shop be placed into the PROPERTIES subsidiary, Susan discussed the profitability of commercial printing businesses with Mark Stanton, president of the Land of Lincoln Printers Association, the state trade organization. Mark pointed out that the average printer in the United States has a profit margin of 5.5 percent, while the average in the Chicago metropolitan area is barely 4 percent.

Return on assets in the industry is 7.5 percent nationwide and 5.2 percent locally.

Estimates regarding the profits that could be earned on commercial sales are far from precise, but the best guess is that in 2010 commercial sales could bring in as much as $40,000 in pretax profits (in 2010 dollars). This amount could increase to $45,000 in 2011 (in 2011 dollars), given more time to advertise and build customer relationships. Although uncertain, the pretax profits that stem from external business are expected to increase by 5 percent per year after 2011, including both volume growth and price inflation. Note that the pretax profit amounts include all costs related to the external printing business except marketing costs, which are estimated at $6,000 in 2010, and are expected to increase at the 3 percent inflation rate.

Finally, the System's purchasing manager has questioned the company's policy regarding external printing contracts: What is the company's current policy, and might a change in policy have a bearing on the decision at hand? The discount rate to use in the analysis has also been an issue under discussion. Susan believes that the discount rate should reflect the divisional placement of the print shop, but some staffers have disagreed with this view. "After all," said one, "the primary factor in choosing a discount rate is the riskiness of the cash flows being discounted."

Assume that you are the administrative resident at Cook County Health System, and you have been given the task of analyzing the print shop situation and recommending a course of action. In assigning the project, your preceptor indicated that a risk analysis was appropriate. When asked for more guidance, his response was, "You know more about this sort of thing than I do. Just do it!"

EXHIBIT 21.1
Cook County Health System: Printing Currently Done by Outside Vendors

	Fiscal Year	
	2008	2009
Graphics Printing		
Mercury	$ 85,002.31	$ 7,727.86
Universal Color Graphics	16,982.44	12,588.00
Windy City Press	9,300.00	24,446.00
Northern Illinois Printing	5,628.50	711.94
Pickett Press	3,526.14	2,337.10
Sir Speedy	1,962.58	8,939.50
Northwest Suburban Printing	85.46	0.00
C & S Printing	1,161.00	0.00
Great Lakes Printing Service	0.00	75,292.83
Total graphics printing	$123,648.43	$132,043.23
90% to be brought in-house	$111,283.59	$118,838.91
Forms Printing		
Continuous	$223,826.43	$239,493.82
Stock tab	77,150.41	82,550.50
Labels	68,032.88	65,965.88
Carbon snap	97,563.27	106,283.44
Envelopes	61,096.52	62,435.89
Lab mount	5,095.35	5,126.33
Flat 1/2 side	42,266.69	40,986.45
Special	39,910.37	46,295.47
Oversize	1,458.19	0.00
Special service	1,190.00	2,743.98
Card stock	21,237.40	23,479.11
NCR flat	21,017.01	22,798.19
Total forms printing	$659,844.52	$698,159.06
30% to be brought in-house	$197,953.36	$209,447.71
Total vendor printing	$783,492.95	$830,202.29
Total to be brought in-house	$309,236.95	$328,286.62

Item	Estimated Cost
Two-color press	$ 65,000
Two-color press (small), Model 9860	26,000
Ten-hole drill press	7,800
Futura F-20 folder system	13,000
Collator-stitcher, 12 bin	28,000
Bookmaker, Michael 1000E	5,300
Camera with processor	14,000
Paper plate, AB Dick 148	11,500
Three-knife trimmer	12,000
Infrared dryer systems (2)	5,000
Delivery van	25,000
Miscellaneous items	5,000
Total capital investment	$217,600

EXHIBIT 21.2
Cook County Health System: Equipment Capital Investment Requirements

Number	Position	Annual Salary
1	Lead printer	$ 42,000
1	Delivery person	25,000
1	Clerical assistant	15,000
	Projected raw-labor expense	$ 82,000
	Plus: 20 percent fringe benefits	16,400
	Total annual incremental labor costs	$ 98,400

EXHIBIT 21.3
Cook County Health System: Print Shop's Incremental Labor Costs (2009 dollars)

ST. JEROME TEACHING HOSPITAL

22

MERGER ANALYSIS

THE PATIENT BASE of Marshland County, Ohio, is currently served by three hospitals: (1) St. Jerome Teaching Hospital, a not-for-profit university-related hospital with 525 beds; (2) Erie Regional Medical Center, a 250-bed for-profit hospital owned by Hospital Associates of America (HAA), a national chain; and (3) Marshland General, a 400-bed, not-for-profit, acute care hospital owned by Buckeye Healthcare. St. Jerome and Marshland are located less than one mile from one another, while Erie Regional is about five miles away from St. Jerome, in a newer and more rapidly developing section of town.

The service area has a total of 1,175 licensed beds, or about 3.5 beds per 1,000 population, which is higher than the national average of about 2.8 beds per 1,000 and much greater than the roughly 2 beds per 1,000 needed under aggressive utilization management. Of course, as a tertiary care facility, St. Jerome receives patients from throughout the state, but the bulk of its patients still come from the local five-county area.

With an excess of hospital beds in the service area, the status quo may not survive the changing healthcare environment. Indeed, Marshland General has had some tough years recently, as evidenced by its number of discharges, which have fallen to 11,412 in 2009 from 12,055 in 2008 and 12,824 in 2007. Additionally, HAA has been aggressive in building market share in other areas of Ohio, both through acquisitions and hospital expansions. With these factors in place, some consolidation in the local hospital market will likely take place, and the most likely result is the acquisition of Marshland General by either St. Jerome or HAA.

Marshland General operated as a county hospital for more than 50 years and hence developed a reputation for providing healthcare services to the poor. After many years of operating losses, the county concluded that it could no longer afford to operate the hospital. So, in 1983, the county sold the hospital for $1 to Buckeye Healthcare, a not-for-profit managed care organization and provider, which by 2009 had become the state's largest integrated healthcare company.

Buckeye Healthcare's major business line is managed care. Its numerous plans, including HMO, PPO, POS, Medicare, and Medicaid, serve more than 800,000 members in 25 Ohio counties, encompassing all of the major metropolitan areas. In addition to managed care plans, Buckeye Healthcare owns nine different providers: two acute care hospitals, including Marshland General; two primary care hospitals; one rehabilitation hospital; one mental health facility; one hospice; one home health care provider; and one retirement facility.

Marshland General is the flagship of Buckeye Healthcare's provider network, and, as such, the company has kept the hospital in excellent condition in spite of falling inpatient utilization. In fact, in recent years, Marshland General has built a new, state-of-the-art HeartCare Center and a modern MaternityCare Center. Furthermore, Marshland General operates a full-service emergency department and a medical helicopter service.

In response to the current situation, St. Jerome has formed a special committee to consider the feasibility of making an offer to Buckeye Healthcare to acquire Marshland General. The committee's primary goals are as follows:

1. To place a dollar value on Marshland General's equity (fund) capital, assuming that the hospital will be acquired and operated by St. Jerome
2. To develop a financing plan for the acquisition

In addition, the committee has been asked to consider two other issues related to the potential acquisition.

1. What is the best organizational structure for a combined enterprise? Currently, both Marshland General

and St. Jerome have separate boards of directors and management staffs. Of course, the senior members of the board of Marshland General currently are Buckeye Healthcare officers.

2. Should the medical staffs of the two hospitals be integrated, and, if so, in what way? The medical staff of Marshland General consists of local physicians, including many family practice physicians, while the medical staff at St. Jerome is almost entirely made up of specialists, and all are members of the local university's College of Medicine with responsibilities that go well beyond clinical practice. A new committee will be formed to finalize recommendations on these issues should St. Jerome's management agree to move forward with the acquisition offer, but some preliminary judgments are sought at this time.

As a starting point in the valuation analysis, the committee has obtained historical income statement and balance sheet data on both hospitals. Exhibit 22.1 contains the data for Marshland General, while Exhibit 22.2 provides the data for St. Jerome. Note that both sets of statements focus on operating data, which are considered to be most relevant to the analysis. In addition, some relevant comparative data are presented in Exhibit 22.3. Finally, relevant market data are contained in Exhibit 22.4. (Note that data in Exhibits 22.3 and 22.4 reflect late-2009 conditions.)

One of the toughest tasks that the committee faces is the development of Marshland General's pro forma (forecasted) cash flow statements, which form the basis of a discounted cash flow valuation. Several basic questions must be answered before any numbers can be generated:

1. What synergies, if any, can be realized from the merger, and how long will it take for any synergies to be realized? For example, can duplications be eliminated? Both hospitals have "mercy flight" helicopters and both offer full emergency department services, even though the two hospitals are only one mile apart. Also, what is the impact of such operational changes

on revenues and costs and hence on the net cash flows that Marshland General's assets can produce?
2. Once the consolidation takes place and all synergies have been realized, what is the long-term growth prospect for Marshland General's cash flows?
3. What impact will the acquisition have on St. Jerome's own cash flows? Any change in St. Jerome's revenues or costs that results from the acquisition must be included in the analysis.

The answers to these questions, and others, form the basis for the pro forma cash flow statements.

Assume that you are the chair of the special committee formed at St. Jerome Teaching Hospital to evaluate the potential acquisition. You must present your findings and recommendations to the hospital's board of directors. Because the case contains far less information than normally available in a merger analysis, especially when the potential merger is friendly, you will be required to make many difficult assumptions to complete your analysis. Although you do not know much about Marshland General's local market, you do know the current trends in the healthcare industry. Use this knowledge to help make judgments about the case. The quality of many, if not most, real-world financial analyses depends more on the validity of the underlying assumptions than on the theoretical "correctness" of the analytical techniques.

Note that there is no preferred solution to this case, so your case analysis will be judged as much on the assumptions used in the analysis as on the analysis itself. Finally, remember that numerous risk-analysis techniques are available that can be used to give decision makers some feel for the risks involved.

EXHIBIT 22.1
Marshland General: Historical Financial Statements (millions of dollars)

	2005	2006	2007	2008	2009
Income Statements:					
Inpatient revenue	$ 81.624	$ 88.249	$ 99.010	$105.332	$110.384
Outpatient revenue	22.861	27.067	34.628	43.616	50.810
Gross patient revenue	$104.485	$115.316	$133.638	$148.948	$161.194
Allowances and discounts	33.699	38.626	44.622	51.198	62.006
Net patient revenue	$ 70.786	$ 76.690	$ 89.016	$ 97.750	$ 99.188
Other operating revenue	1.922	1.515	1.367	1.725	1.048
Total operating revenue	$ 72.708	$ 78.205	$ 90.383	$ 99.475	$100.236
Patient services expenses	$ 60.245	$ 73.858	$ 81.525	$ 90.645	$ 89.505
Interest expense	3.045	3.147	3.093	3.002	2.980
Depreciation	3.466	3.689	4.395	4.258	6.031
Total operating expense	$ 66.756	$ 80.694	$ 89.013	$ 97.905	$ 98.516
Net income	$ 5.952	($ 2.489)	$ 1.370	$ 1.570	$ 1.720
Balance Sheets:					
Cash and investments	$ 2.388	$ 1.538	$ 0.162	$ 0.185	$ 0.198
Accounts receivable	18.860	20.581	20.821	21.570	16.732
Other current assets	4.539	8.475	4.669	2.585	2.898
Total current assets	$ 25.787	$ 30.594	$ 25.652	$ 24.340	$ 19.828
Gross plant and equipment	$102.596	$116.694	$122.611	$133.499	$146.130
Accumulated depreciation	27.243	30.505	34.900	39.158	45.189
Net plant and equipment	$ 75.353	$ 86.189	$ 87.711	$ 94.341	$100.941
Total assets	$101.140	$116.783	$113.363	$118.681	$120.769
Current liabilities	$ 9.182	$ 13.584	$ 5.771	$ 10.689	$ 11.431
Long-term debt	33.572	47.302	50.325	49.155	48.781
Total liabilities	$ 42.754	$ 60.886	$ 56.096	$ 59.844	$ 60.212
Fund balance	58.386	55.897	57.267	58.837	60.557
Total claims	$101.140	$116.783	$113.363	$118.681	$120.769

EXHIBIT 22.2
St. Jerome Teaching Hospital: Historical Financial Statements (millions of dollars)

	2005	2006	2007	2008	2009
Income Statements:					
Inpatient revenue	$238.510	$287.559	$328.047	$363.236	$398.997
Outpatient revenue	47.963	57.351	69.252	89.992	103.746
Gross patient revenue	$286.473	$344.910	$397.299	$453.228	$502.743
Allowances and discounts	82.053	107.256	128.645	170.058	185.301
Net patient revenue	$204.420	$237.654	$268.654	$283.170	$317.442
Other operating revenue	5.587	8.899	12.193	22.672	9.979
Total operating revenue	$210.007	$246.553	$280.847	$305.842	$327.421
Patient services expenses	$178.788	$207.596	$231.673	$254.704	$277.938
Interest expense	9.232	10.468	11.983	10.691	9.997
Depreciation	13.289	16.637	19.621	23.286	26.489
Total operating expense	$201.309	$234.701	$263.277	$288.681	$314.424
Net income	$ 8.698	$ 11.852	$ 17.570	$ 17.161	$ 12.997
Balance Sheets:					
Cash and investments	$ 17.918	$ 19.862	$ 24.660	$ 27.726	$ 25.220
Accounts receivable	66.212	72.989	99.867	100.297	97.494
Other current assets	12.315	16.771	20.741	20.542	22.757
Total current assets	$ 96.445	$109.622	$145.268	$148.565	$145.471
Gross plant and equipment	$348.288	$341.064	$335.313	$362.152	$400.546
Accumulated depreciation	75.139	76.575	90.056	109.468	123.567
Net plant and equipment	$273.149	$264.489	$245.257	$252.684	$276.979
Total assets	$369.594	$374.111	$390.525	$401.249	$422.450
Current liabilities	$ 42.437	$ 35.061	$ 39.511	$ 37.733	$ 39.817
Long-term debt	146.997	147.038	141.432	136.773	142.893
Total liabilities	$189.434	$182.099	$180.943	$174.506	$182.710
Fund balance	180.160	192.012	209.582	226.743	239.740
Total claims	$369.594	$374.111	$390.525	$401.249	$422.450

Note: The hospital's current target cash balance is $5 million.

	Marshland	St. Jerome
Average age of plant	6.8 years	8.5 years
Licensed beds	400	525
Occupancy rate	52.7%	64.2%
Average length of stay	5.5 days	6.6 days
Number of discharges	11,412	19,748
Medicare percent	57.2%	29.7%
Medicaid percent	10.3%	13.0%
Medicare case mix index	1.51	2.13
Gross price per discharge	$11,688	$20,204
Net price per discharge	$5,850	$12,757
Cost per discharge	$5,703	$12,144

EXHIBIT 22.3 Selected Comparative Data

U.S. Treasury Yield Curve:

Maturity	Interest Rate
6 months	3.0%
1 year	3.5
5 years	3.9
10 years	4.5
20 years	5.0
30 years	5.1

Market Risk Premium:

Historical risk premium	7.0%
Average current risk premium as forecasted by three investment banking firms	6.0%

Market Betas, Capitalization, and Tax Rates of Two Publicly Traded Hospital Companies:

Company	Beta	Debt/Asset Ratio	Tax Rate
Provident Healthcare	1.1	50%	40%
National Health Company	1.2	65%	43%

EXHIBIT 22.4 Selected Market and Hospital Data

EXHIBIT 22.4 (continued) Selected Market and Hospital Data

Ratio of Stock Price to EBITDA per Share:

Provident Healthcare	6.1
National Health Company	7.9

Ratio of Total Equity Market Value to Number of Discharges:

Provident Healthcare	$7,000
National Health Company	$6,000

Proportion of Cash to Current Assets:

Large hospital average	5.0%

EBITDA: earnings before interest, taxes, depreciation, and amortization

Note: The data in this table reflect assumptions, as opposed to actual data, to ease the case analysis.

SOUTH BEACH HEALTH PARTNERS

23

JOINT VENTURE ANALYSIS

SOUTH BEACH HOSPITAL (the Hospital) is a 320-bed, acute care, not-for-profit hospital located in Miami Beach, Florida. It is well known as a leader in new technology and hence draws patients from as far away as Palm Beach to the north and Key West to the south. The Hospital contracts with the Gold Coast Radiology Group (the Group) to provide radiology services for its patients. Basically, the Hospital furnishes the radiology equipment and technicians and performs the tests, while the physicians in the Group "read" the results. Because the Group bills patients separately for the readings, no direct payment is made from the Hospital to the Group.

Assume it is now 1988. At the end of one of the monthly medical staff meetings, Dr. Warren Berg, head of the Group, presented a proposal to Mark Covaleski, the Hospital's chief executive officer. The Group wants to form a partnership with the Hospital to purchase a biliary lithotripter, a device that uses shock waves to crush gallstones. Lithotripsy emerged in the early 1980s as a noninvasive way to shatter kidney stones: Patients are placed in a water bath, partially anesthetized, and then subjected to repeated focused blasts of shock waves transmitted through the water. By 1988, renal lithotripsy was well developed, and researchers were beginning to apply the same technology to gallstones, which are extremely common and affect about 20 million Americans. With about 300,000 cholecystectomies (surgical removal of the gallbladder) performed annually, biliary lithotripsy offers the prospect of a painless, noninvasive, and cost-saving alternative to surgery.

The biliary lithotripter, which costs about $1 million, has not yet received approval from the Food and Drug Administration (FDA), and hence it does not qualify for Medicare/Medicaid reimbursement. However, the FDA has granted approval to begin clinical trials. If these trials satisfy the FDA standards for efficacy and safety, the biliary lithotripter manufacturers will be permitted to freely market the technology. (For more information on the approval process, see the FDA website at www.fda.gov.) The Group will be involved in lithotripter usage because radiologists must read the ultrasound images that are used to locate the stones and confirm that the treatment has been effective.

Mark had recently read an article on biliary lithotripsy, and he is supportive of the idea. Furthermore, Dr. Berg mentioned that he had talked to the president of Medical Equipment International (MEI), one of the biliary lithotripter manufacturers. During the conversation, MEI promised to give the Hospital exclusive purchase rights in its service area during the trial period, which is a process expected to take about two years.

The idea of being an exclusive provider of gallstone lithotripsy appeals to Mark, even if it only lasts for two years. First, by offering this procedure, the Hospital is reinforcing its position as the regional leader in new technology. Second, an early start will position the Hospital as the leading provider if the technology becomes available to competing hospitals. Mark does not believe that the Hospital's board of trustees will be willing to bear the entire risk of the purchase, but he thinks that they might be willing to go along with a joint venture. Thus, Mark asked Dr. Berg to look into the matter further and develop a specific joint venture proposal.

Mark had almost forgotten the matter when, two months later, Dr. Berg appeared with the following proposal: (Exhibit 23.1 contains a summary of the proposed financing.)

1. A separate business entity, South Beach Health Partners (the Partnership), will be formed.
2. The Partnership will have two general partners: the Group and the Hospital. The Group will put up $300,000 in capital and retain 60 percent management control, while the Hospital will furnish $200,000 in capital and obtain 40 percent control. (The Group is incorporated, but it files federal income taxes as

an S corporation. It would incorporate a subsidiary S corporation for the sole purpose of investing in the Partnership. S corporations pay no federal income taxes. Rather, as in a partnership, the income is constructively prorated among the owners and taxed as ordinary income.)

3. Twenty-five limited partnerships will be offered to local physicians for $20,000 each. The limited partners (the LPs) will have no liability beyond their $20,000 investments but, on the other hand, will have no control rights. (The Partnership is purposely restricted to 25 limited partners because a larger number will require a more complicated partnership registration procedure with the State of Florida.)

4. An additional $1 million will be obtained from the Miami National Bank in the form of a five-year term (amortized) loan carrying an interest rate of 8 percent. The bank will require the Partnership to pledge the equipment as collateral for the loan. In the event of default by the Partnership, the market value of the equipment will be used first to offset the principal balance, and then the Group will be liable for 60 percent and the Hospital for 40 percent of any remaining balance.

The $2 million initial capital infusion will be just sufficient to purchase and install the lithotripter and to pay the consulting, legal, and accounting costs associated with forming the Partnership. The Hospital will lease the Partnership the space for the lithotripter, furnish the technical support required to operate the equipment, and handle billing and collections. Of course, all services provided to the Partnership by the Hospital will be handled at arm's length, and hence the Partnership will pay the Hospital prevailing market rates for the services provided.

The Partnership itself will not be taxed, but its distributions represent income and hence will be taxed on the basis of each partner's tax status. The distributions to the Hospital will be nontaxable because the joint venture is consistent with the Hospital's not-for-profit status. The distributions to the Group and to the LPs will be taxed as ordinary income. However, about 50 percent of the distributions will represent a return of capital (depreciation cash flow), which is not taxed, and hence taxable investors will pay taxes at an effective rate of only about 20 percent.

The cash flows from the Partnership will be distributed according to the following plan:

1. The Partnership will distribute all earned net cash flow to the partners at the end of each year.
2. At the end of the first year, the general partners will receive 30 percent of the cash flow and the LPs will receive 70 percent. Following the distribution at the end of each year, the total accumulated dollar return provided to the LPs will be calculated. If this amount is less than the LPs' total contribution, the LPs will continue to receive 70 percent of the cash flow in the following year.
3. In the years succeeding the year in which the LPs recover their initial contribution, 50 percent of the cash flow will be distributed to the general partners, while 50 percent will go to the LPs.
4. The cash flow allocated to the general partners will be distributed proportionally to the Group and to the Hospital on the basis of each partner's relative contribution: 60 percent will go to the Group and 40 percent to the Hospital.

Of course, the key to a sound financial analysis is good cash flow estimates. Mark and Dr. Berg devoted an entire day to the cash flow estimation process, and many other individuals provided input. If the joint venture gets off the ground, the lithotripter will be in operation by the end of the year (Year 0). The equipment will be available for 50 weeks each year, and the best estimate is that four procedures will be performed per week during the first year (Year 1).

Although the lithotripter is only approved for trials, several third-party payers have expressed an interest in supporting the testing. If the technology is successful, biliary lithotripsy will significantly lower future costs for the treatment of gallstones. Based on discussions with selected payers, the Partnership is expected to receive $5,000 per procedure on average. Thus, the net revenue in Year 1 is forecasted to be 4(50)($5,000) = $1,000,000. Physician and public awareness will increase after the first year, and hence volume is projected to increase to five procedures per week during Year 2. Although FDA approval will mean additional utilization by Medicare/Medicaid patients in Year 3, at least one competing hospital will likely have its own lithotripter at this time. Thus, volume is expected to fall back to four procedures per week in Year 3, to three procedures per week in Year 4, and to two procedures per week in Year 5.

Projecting the trend for net revenue per procedure is difficult. On the one hand, it might be possible to increase the charge for biliary lithotripsy by the overall inflation rate, or even more. But on the other hand, FDA approval will mean that Medicare/Medicaid patients will join the patient mix, and these payments often are set below the standard charge; indeed, such payments could be below costs. Because these factors tend to offset one another, no inflation adjustments will be applied to charge estimates.

Technology is moving quickly in this area, so assessing whether the lithotripter will have an economic life of more than five years is difficult. For the same reason, estimating the machine's salvage value at the end of five years is also difficult. Because of the uncertainties involved, Mark and Dr. Berg agreed to assume a five-year life for the Partnership and a zero salvage value for the equipment.

Exhibit 23.2 contains the forecasted cash flow statements for the Partnership for Years 1 and 2. Note the following points:

1. Technician costs are estimated at $50 per procedure, so total technician support for Year 1 is (4)(50)$50 = $10,000.
2. Clerical costs are estimated at $15 per procedure, so total clerical expense for Year 1 is (4)(50)$15 = $3,000.
3. Technician and clerical salaries are expected to increase at an annual rate of 5 percent.
4. Rent, insurance, and marketing expenses are forecasted to be $15,000, $10,000, and $5,000, respectively, in Year 1. These costs are expected to increase at the projected inflation rate of 5 percent.
5. Expendable supplies are estimated to cost $20 per procedure, and hence the Year 1 total supplies cost is

(4)(50)$20 = $4,000. Further, the cost of expendables is expected to increase at the 5 percent inflation rate.

6. The service contract on the lithotripter is expected to cost $50,000 in Years 1 and 2, $75,000 in Years 3 and 4, and $100,000 in Year 5. These costs increase over time because cumulative usage increases the need for maintenance and parts replacement.

7. The Partnership will have to pay property taxes on the equipment, currently estimated to be $23,000 in Year 1, $24,000 in Year 2, $25,000 in Year 3, $26,000 in Year 4, and $27,000 in Year 5.

8. The Partnership's administrative expenses are estimated to be $30,000 per year. These expenses consist of accounting and legal fees as well as reimbursement for management time spent on Partnership business. These costs are expected to increase at the 5 percent inflation rate.

9. Principal and interest expenses are based on annual amortization of an 8 percent, five-year loan of $1 million.

10. Miscellaneous expenses, which consist of the costs involved in the semiannual partners meeting, forms printing, expendable clerical supplies, and so on, are expected to be a constant $20,000 over the next five years.

Mark and Dr. Berg are most concerned about the estimates for weekly volume, and hence they spent a great deal of time developing the following data:

	Weekly Volume				
Case	Year 1	Year 2	Year 3	Year 4	Year 5
Worst	3	4	3	2	1
Most likely	4	5	4	3	2
Best	5	6	5	4	3

These estimates assume that the biliary lithotripter will meet the manufacturer's expectations regarding efficacy and safety. However, any problems in this regard could mean that the trials could be curtailed or even discontinued. Even if the trials were completed, failure to obtain final FDA approval will mean a whole new ball game. **Assuming no problems during the trial and subsequent FDA approval,** the best estimates for the probabilities of the above scenarios are 25 percent for the best and worst cases and 50 percent for the most likely case.

The current yield on 20-year T-bonds is 5 percent. Furthermore, a local brokerage firm estimated the market risk premium to be 5 percentage points. Thus, according to the Capital Asset Pricing Model (CAPM), the current required rate of return on an average-risk (large publicly traded company with a beta equal to 1.0) stock investment is 10 percent.

In addition to the efficacy concerns, all parties have expressed concern over two other issues. First, are there any indirect costs or benefits (i.e., costs or benefits that do not appear in the estimated cash flows) to any of the parties to the venture? Second, does the Partnership raise any legal or ethical issues for any of the parties?

Assume that you have been hired as a consultant to examine the feasibility of the proposed joint venture. You must assess the situation and prepare a report for the Hospital and the Group. Mark and Dr. Berg know that the joint venture will never be successful unless all parties are satisfied with the financial arrangements. Thus, they believe that an impartial analysis should be conducted to assess the risk/return potential for each party. Furthermore, if any of the parties do not appear to be treated fairly under the initial proposal, they seek recommendations that will increase overall fairness and hence give the proposal a better chance of success.

In beginning your analysis, you recognize that several different cash flow/discount rate formats are available for valuing businesses. In essence, the partnership analysis is merely business valuation but from the perspective of different classes of equity participants. To allow the analysis to include multiple equity perspectives, it is necessary to structure the cash flows using the free-cash-flow-to-equityholders method. Here, the focus is on the cash flows that are available for distribution to equityholders, so interest expense (and any other creditor flows) must be subtracted from the cash flow stream. (Note that this format differs from a typical capital budgeting analysis, in which debt flows are not considered.) Because the estimated net cash flows are equity flows,

178   *Cases in Healthcare Finance*

they must be discounted by a cost of equity. (Typical capital budgeting cash flows are operating cash flows and hence are discounted by the differential risk-adjusted corporate cost of capital.)

You also note that sensitivity analysis is not useful in this situation because the unique cash flow distribution system confounds such an analysis. Also, internal rate of return, although useful for the base case, breaks down in a scenario analysis because some scenarios create non-normal cash flows. Thus, you plan to use standard scenario-analysis techniques for your risk analysis with net present value as the profitability measure. Furthermore, because the purpose of scenario analysis is to assess risk, rather than incorporate it, you plan to use a constant 15 percent discount rate for all partners in the scenario analysis.

Finally, you can't seem to shake the feeling that something might go wrong during the clinical trials. In fact, a nurse that had worked as a clinical consultant for MEI before moving to Miami has expressed some concern about the effectiveness of biliary lithotripsy. "Lithotripsy may work well on kidney stones, but I'll bet you a dollar to a doughnut that it won't work on gallstones," she was reported to say. Thus, you want to ensure that the analysis considers at least one scenario that recognizes that the technology might fail to produce the desired results.

Exhibit 23.1
South Beach
Health Partners:
Partnership
Financing Summary

Capital Contribution	General Partners	Limited Partners	Debt Financing
$ 300,000	Group		
200,000	Hospital		
500,000		25 @ $20,000 each	
1,000,000			Miami NB
$ 2,000,000			

EXHIBIT 23.2
South Beach Health Partners: Forecasted Cash Flow Statements

	Year 1	Year 2
Net revenues	$1,000,000	$1,250,000
Cash operating costs:		
Technician support	$ 10,000	$ 13,125
Clerical support	3,000	3,938
Rent	15,000	15,750
Insurance	10,000	10,500
Marketing expenses	5,000	5,250
Expendable supplies	4,000	5,250
Service contract	50,000	50,000
Property taxes	23,000	24,000
Administrative expense	30,000	31,500
Principal repayment	170,456	184,093
Interest expense	80,000	66,363
Miscellaneous expenses	20,000	20,000
Total expenses	$ 420,456	$ 429,769
Partnership net cash flow	$ 579,544	$ 820,231

BLOOMINGTON CLINICS
PRACTICE VALUATION

24

BLOOMINGTON CLINICS (the Practice), a medical group practice in Bloomington, Illinois, operates two walk-in clinics. (For more information on physician group practices, see the American Medical Group Association website at www.amga.org or the Medical Group Management Association website at www.mgma.org.) The Practice consists of five physicians—three are board certified in family practice and two are certified in internal medicine. Of the five, three work full time, while the remaining two work half-time, resulting in four full-time equivalent (FTE) physicians. The Practice is organized as a for-profit corporation, but for tax purposes the business is classified as an S corporation. (In an S corporation, the business pays no taxes. Rather, the corporation's taxable income is constructively distributed to the owners, who pay personal taxes on the income.)

The Practice was founded ten years ago by two physicians (the part timers) who wanted to have more free time than their solo practices allowed. Initially, the Practice had only one location, but a second was recently added. The downtown clinic, whose patients predominantly come directly from work sites, is open Monday through Friday from 8 a.m. to 2 p.m. The midtown clinic, whose patients mostly come from home, is open Monday through Saturday from 8 a.m. to 8 p.m. Exhibit 24.1 provides basic utilization and payer data for the two clinics. With the current medical and clerical staffs, as well as clinic space, the Practice's patient volume can grow as much as 50 percent without the need for additional personnel or facilities.

The five physicians who make up the Practice own the business. However, the two founding physicians control the business: each has a 35 percent ownership stake. The remaining three physicians each owns 10 percent of the business. Because the controlling physicians are looking to fully retire in the near future, they would like to sell the business. The remaining owners are less enthusiastic about selling out, but as minority owners their alternatives are limited.

Preliminary work by a business broker has identified several potential buyers, including another for-profit physician group, a wealthy individual investor, and a local not-for-profit hospital. However, the Practice's owners do not want to enter into any negotiations without first obtaining an independent appraisal of the business.

The most recent income statement of the business is contained in Exhibit 24.2. Note that the statement is based on an assumed effective average tax rate of 20 percent, which is the rate applicable if the Practice were to file as a C corporation. However, the tax rate that must be applied in any valuation is the marginal tax rate of the acquirer. A condensed balance sheet was prepared for the purpose of this appraisal and is contained in Exhibit 24.3. The Practice plans to maintain the current debt ratio into the foreseeable future and has an agreement with a lending institution to borrow funds at a rate of 8 percent. In addition to assets used in the day-to-day operations of the business, the Practice holds nonoperating assets (marketable securities and investment properties). The marketable securities represent a "rainy day" fund, while the investment properties were acquired to diversify the asset holdings and revenue stream of the Practice.

Of course, the value of the Practice is not a function of past cash flows but of future cash flows. Heidi Wilde, the administrator of Bloomington Clinics, was given the task of estimating the business's future cash flows. The first thing she did was to estimate the expected revenue growth rates for the next five years; these estimates are contained in Exhibit 24.4. Because of the uncertainty inherent in future volume estimates, and hence in revenue growth rates, three scenarios are presented. Although Heidi wanted to attach differential probabilities to the three scenarios, her best guess is that one scenario is as likely as the others. Regardless of the near-term revenue growth scenario, the Practice's long-term, sustainable growth rate (Year 6 and beyond) is expected to be 5 percent.

In terms of costs, the Practice's cost structure listed in the notes to Exhibit 24.2 is expected to hold in the immediate future, with fixed costs (including depreciation) increasing at a 5 percent annual rate. Furthermore, the Practice will have to invest roughly $15,000 each year (in Year 1 dollars) in new equipment under the most likely growth scenario, $20,000 under the higher growth scenario, and $10,000 under the lower growth scenario. Inflation is expected to increase these capital investment amounts by 5 percent per year.

Assume that you have been hired as an independent appraiser to place a value on the business. To use the discounted cash flow (DCF) approach, it will be necessary to estimate the required rate of return on an equity investment in the Practice. Little market data are available for guidance, but the current yield on long-term Treasury bonds is 6 percent, while the historical risk premium on the market, which reflects the premium on an average-risk common stock investment, is about 5 to 7 percent. Of course, there are significant risk and liquidity differences between direct ownership of a relatively small group practice and ownership of the stock of a large, publicly traded corporation. To complicate the valuation even more, control issues could arise in direct ownership.

In addition to the DCF approach, numerous other techniques for valuing small businesses are available. Two methods commonly applied to value medical practices are variants of the market multiple approach, in which some proxy for value—for example, earnings—is multiplied by a market-determined factor that best expresses the relationship of that proxy to equity value. For this appraisal, you have determined that recent purchases of family physician practices have been priced at 1.8 to 2.2 times projected revenue and (more roughly) at $800,000 to $1,000,000 times the number of FTE physicians in the Practice.

With this information at hand, your task is to place a value on the Practice. In addition, the majority owners of the Practice have asked you to comment on the following issues:

1. Does the valuation depend on who will make the acquisition? For example, would a not-for-profit hospital place a different value on the Practice than would another for-profit group practice? If so, what factors drive this differential?

2. If the valuation methods do not result in consistent values for any acquirer, explain (a) why the differences exist and (b) which method is the most reliable.
3. Is there any difference in the per share values of the 35 percent ownership of the two founders as opposed to the 10 percent ownership of each of the other three physicians?
4. How does the fact that the Practice uses debt financing affect the analysis, if at all? Does the presence of financial leverage make the Practice a more or less attractive acquisition candidate?
5. Will there be a productivity problem if the Practice is acquired? That is, will the remaining (and potentially newly hired) physicians be as productive when they are employees of the Practice as they were (and would be) as owners?
6. Assuming that the acquirer will make an initial offer below your valuation, can you recommend a negotiation strategy that will help the owners settle at the highest possible acquisition price?

EXHIBIT 24.1
Bloomington Clinics: Utilization and Payer Data

Average Number of Visits by Day:

	Downtown	Midtown
Monday	39	57
Tuesday	33	46
Wednesday	33	43
Thursday	34	44
Friday	33	28
Saturday	—	37
Total	172	255

Payer Breakdown:

	Downtown	Midtown
Employer	27.9%	12.5%
Cash/Credit card	25.7	35.7
Blue Shield	20.9	24.4
Commercial	14.5	18.8
Medicare	11.0	8.6
Total	100.0%	100.0%

EXHIBIT 24.2
Bloomington Clinics: Historical Income Statement

Net revenues	$1,491,791
Operating expenses	1,069,076
EBIT	$ 422,715
Interest expense	25,575
EBT	$ 397,140
Taxes	79,428
Net profit	$ 317,712

EBIT: earnings before interest and tax; EBT: earnings before tax

Notes:
1. Operating expenses include depreciation of 11,070.
2. At these levels of income, the Practice's effective tax rate (if taxed as a C corporation) is about 20 percent.
3. Operating expenses consist of a fixed component plus a variable component. The best estimates for this year are a fixed component of 719,997 and a variable component of $349,079. Thus, the current variable operating expenses expressed as a percentage of net revenues is 23.4 percent.
4. Capital expenditures for the year were $15,000.

EXHIBIT 24.3
Bloomington Clinics: Condensed Balance Sheet

ASSETS:	
Cash and cash equivalents	$ 73,475
Marketable securities	42,399
Accounts receivable	85,702
Medical and administrative supplies	9,890
Current assets	$ 211,466
Net plant and equipment	1,689,524
Investment properties	450,461
Total assets	$2,351,451
LIABILITIES AND OWNER'S EQUITY:	
Notes payable	$ 352,718
Owner's equity	1,998,733
Total liabilities and equity	$2,351,451

Note: Adjustments to the amount of debt in the capital structure occur at year end. Thus, interest expense on the income statement can be calculated from the previous year's balance of notes payable.

EXHIBIT 24.4
Revenue Growth Rate Estimates

Case	Year 1	Year 2	Year 3	Year 4	Year 5
Best	11.0%	9.0%	8.0%	7.0%	6.0%
Most likely	9.0	8.0	7.0	6.0	5.0
Worst	7.0	6.0	5.0	5.0	5.0

25
UNIVERSITY FACULTY PRACTICE
PHYSICIAN EXTENDER ANALYSIS

UNIVERSITY FACULTY PRACTICE (the Practice) is the not-for-profit corporation that controls the clinical operations of the medical faculty of Shasta University. The Practice provides all physician services for Shasta Health System (the System), which consists of six hospitals plus supporting services that, in total, provide the entire continuum of care. The main inpatient facility is a 650-bed tertiary care academic medical center, although the System also owns two rural 50-bed hospitals, two 125-bed community hospitals, and a 250-bed long-term-care facility. In addition to inpatient facilities, the System has several outpatient clinics and centers.

The Practice's vice president for outpatient services, Dr. Paul Phillips, is exploring the use of physician extenders in the clinics as a way of enhancing physician productivity and, ultimately, the Practice's profitability. As a start, three clinics are being targeted for evaluation: the outpatient surgery pre-op and post-op clinic, the internal medicine (family practice) clinic, and the eldercare clinic.

In recent years, the role of physician extenders has evolved to the point where they have a considerable impact on the delivery of care in many different settings. For example, physician extenders can perform more than 80 percent of primary care physicians' patient care duties, including taking medical histories; performing physical examinations; diagnosing and treating illnesses; ordering and interpreting laboratory tests; and, in most situations, prescribing medications.

The use of extenders allows physicians to treat more and higher-acuity patients, therefore expediting patient flow and increasing revenues. Also, because compensation for physician extenders is less than that for physicians, costs per patient visit can be lowered. In addition to the obvious productivity and economic benefits, studies indicate that patient satisfaction improves when physician extenders are used. In essence, they are willing (and able) to spend more time with each patient than physicians typically do. This extra attention often results in better quality of care (real or perceived) and higher patient satisfaction.

However, as the role of physician extenders expanded, it was inevitable that some conflicts would arise. The increasing recognition by third-party payers that extenders are as acceptable as physicians in providing many services means extenders are a potential source of direct competition for physicians, especially in hospital settings where nonphysician executives generally call the shots. Still, physicians at many solo and group practices are using extenders to supplement and complement their work. Conversely, a "hard core" of private practice physicians remains who view extenders as a threat to their gatekeeper position within the healthcare system.

The two primary types of physician extenders are advanced registered nurse practitioners (ARNPs or NPs) and physician assistants (PAs). Although NPs and PAs often perform similar tasks, significant differences do exist. NPs must be licensed in the state in which they practice. To acquire such licensure, an individual must first be licensed as a registered nurse (RN), then meet additional education and practicum requirements that generally lead to a master's degree, and finally pass a national certification examination in one of several specialized areas. (For more information on NPs, see the website of the American Academy of Nurse Practitioners at www.aanp.org.)

PAs must graduate from an accredited physician assistant educational program and then obtain certification by the National Commission on Certification of Physician Assistants. The educational training for a PA is similar to that of a physician, but much shorter—historically only two years. Although PA programs traditionally offered either associate or bachelor's degrees, most programs today are at the master's level. (For more information on PAs, see the website of the American Academy of Physician Assistants at www.aapa.org.)

Although it may appear on the surface that NPs and PAs are perfect substitutes for one another, the differences in educational background create differences in philosophies of care. Because NPs follow the nursing model of care, which focuses on health education and counseling as well as disease prevention, they typically have a special concern for the overall health and welfare of patients. Furthermore, NPs often specialize in particular areas of patient care such as anesthesiology, pediatrics, and women's health. PAs, on the other hand, generally follow the medical model of care, which focuses on diagnosis and treatment. Of course, these are generalizations that do not necessarily apply to specific individuals.

The practice status of physician extenders has been, in large part, driven by state law. Historically, some states allowed NPs to practice independently, while others mandated some physician involvement (collaborative or supervisory). With PAs, most states required that a physician be physically present (or electronically available) when a PA treats a patient. In addition, many states allowed NPs to prescribe all medications independent of physician supervision, while the ability of PAs to prescribe medications was much more limited. However, the Balanced Budget Act of 1997 removed many of the limitations imposed by individual states. Now, both NPs and PAs are allowed to practice without the immediate availability of a supervising physician. Note, however, that NPs are allowed to practice under their own licenses, while PAs must practice under the license of a physician.

The reimbursement of physician extenders, like all reimbursement for healthcare services, is complicated by the fact that many third-party payers use different payment methodologies. For purposes of this case, assume that all payers use the same system as Medicare, which recognizes several different situations in which extenders provide services.

In general, Medicare pays extenders in all settings 85 percent of the physician's fee schedule. Thus, if an extender provided a service that results in a $100 payment to a physician, the payment is $85. However, there are two exceptions to this rule:

1. If the extender and physician both see the patient during an office visit, the combined work of both the extender and physician is reimbursed at 100 percent of the physician fee schedule. However, if the patient service is a procedure (as opposed to a visit) and the work is done primarily by the extender, the 85 percent rule applies.

2. Extenders are paid at a 100 percent rate if the service provided is "incident to" a previous visit or service provided by a physician. This provision requires that the physician be physically on site and that the service provided by the extender is related to a diagnosis made earlier by a physician. Note that "incident to" billing only applies to services provided in offices and clinics as opposed to services provided in hospitals.

In effect, these rules mean that the majority of extender billings in offices and clinics is at the 100 percent rate, so the average extender reimbursement falls somewhere between 85 and 100 percent of the physician rate.

The impact of extenders on physician costs and revenues is highly variable. After some acclimation time, which is required for the extender to become fully productive, several financial impacts are realized:

1. The physician becomes more productive (sees more patients) because the extender can provide the service for a portion of the visit that is billed by the physician. On average nationwide, this increase in the number of billed visits by the physician is estimated to be 10 to 15 percent.
2. The physician's average reimbursement amount increases because the extender is handling the less complex cases. The national average impact on average physician billing amount is estimated at 5 to 10 percent.
3. The extender can see patients independently and bill for those services. On average, extenders see 10 to 20 percent fewer patients than do physicians. Also, because some of these visits are joint with the physician and billed by the physician, the extender can only bill for the remaining visits, which represent 85 to 90 percent of the visits.

Of course, the extent to which these synergies are realized depends on demand (volume). The greater the demand for physician services, the faster an extender can become fully productive and the greater the impact on physician productivity and reimbursement amounts.

As the first step in the decision process regarding the use of physician extenders by the Practice, Dr. Phillips developed the selected data regarding each clinic's physician staffing, productivity, revenues, and costs shown in Exhibit 25.1. For example, the outpatient surgery pre-op and post-op clinic has 2.5 physician FTEs who handle 7,560 patient visits annually that generate $842,481 of revenue (collections). Annual compensation for the physician FTEs totals $485,000.

Assume that you have been hired as a consultant by the Practice to look into the use of physician extenders. Specifically, Dr. Phillips has asked you to (1) estimate the financial impact of using one physician extender at each of the three clinics and (2) recommend the type of extender most appropriate for each setting. (**These tasks are not trivial and might require assumptions and information to supplement the data presented in the case.**)

As a start, you conclude that the national financial-impact data presented earlier must be modified to reflect the actual impact on physician productivity in the three settings. Next, you plan to estimate how many additional visits might be generated at each clinic if one extender is employed. Then, the impact on costs and revenues must be examined. Of course, it might be possible to use an extender to reduce the number of physician FTEs rather than to increase volume. This outcome should be explored if appropriate. Regarding physician extender costs, annual compensation for both NPs and PAs falls into the $60,000 to $80,000 range, depending on geographic location, clinical setting, and work experience.

One of the keys to the analysis is an estimate of the volumes that could be realized at each clinic should an extender be added. Unfortunately, Dr. Phillips has only anecdotal evidence (speculation) on future demand. The best estimate is that patient volume at the outpatient surgery pre-op and post-op clinic is increasing at a 15 percent annual rate as outpatient surgery volume increases. The situation at the internal medicine clinic is quite different. Currently, scheduling has a several-month backlog, and hence a physician extender could be fully used in a relatively short time. Finally, volume at the eldercare clinic has been sporadic and growing slowly, so there is some doubt about whether another clinician is needed.

192 Cases in Healthcare Finance

Dr. Phillips recognizes that you are working with a minimum amount of hard data. Thus, you must make the assumptions used in your analysis clear and supportable.

EXHIBIT 25.1
University Faculty Practice: Selected Data for Three Outpatient Clinics

Outpatient Surgery Pre- and Post-Op Clinic:

Physician FTEs	2.5
Physician costs	$485,000
Physician fees (collections)	$842,481
Daily patient utilization	36
Number of days per week	5
Number of weeks per year	42
Annual patient utilization	7,560
Number of visits per physician	3,024

Internal Medicine (Family Practice) Clinic:

Physician FTEs	2.0
Physician costs	$273,500
Physician fees (collections)	$523,290
Daily patient utilization	30
Number of days per week	4
Number of weeks per year	46
Annual patient utilization	5,520
Number of visits per physician	2,760

Eldercare Clinic:

Physician FTEs	2.25
Physician costs	$335,000
Physician fees (collections)	$454,219
Daily patient utilization	23
Number of days per week	4
Number of weeks per year	48
Annual patient utilization	4,416
Number of visits per physician	1,963

Note: Most physicians in the Practice receive compensation from the University in addition to the amounts listed in this table.

JOHNSON MEMORIAL HOSPITAL
26
COMPETING TECHNOLOGIES WITH BACKFILL

JOHNSON MEMORIAL HOSPITAL (the Hospital) is an 800-bed, acute care, not-for-profit teaching hospital affiliated with one of the largest public universities in the country. In addition to serving the primary and secondary clinical care needs of the neighboring population, the Hospital serves as a tertiary and quaternary referral center for the entire region. For the most part, referred patients seek specialty care that requires unique and often costly clinical expertise and treatment that is available only at select institutions. Thus, it is not surprising that specialty care programs provide the Hospital with about 75 percent of its net operating income.

The Hospital's Center for Digestive Disorders (the Center) is one of the most successful of the specialty care programs. It consistently ranks among the best programs in the country in the diagnosis and treatment of disorders of the gastrointestinal tract. The Center's excellent reputation is further evidenced by the extent of its research funding and its ability to attract patients outside the immediate service area.

The 20 gastroenterologists who staff the Center are physicians drawn from the faculty of the university's College of Medicine. Unlike private practitioners, who focus exclusively on the clinical care of patients, faculty physicians pursue a tripartite mission of clinical service, research, and teaching. It is the successful combination of these pursuits that has helped elevate the status of the Center.

The Center provides care that ranges from gastrointestinal screening to the diagnosis and therapy of common and rare disorders to the referral of appropriate patients to faculty surgeons for the treatment of benign and malignant diseases. The Center encompasses three separate business units: an outpatient clinic, a hospital-based endoscopy suite, and a hospital-based motility (movement) laboratory. Each business unit operates as a separate profit center, and hence each unit maintains its own budget. However, from a patient perspective the care provided is seamless because the Hospital's patient management system expedites patient flow among the Center's three units as well as to outpatient surgery or inpatient status when required.

Although the motility lab generates less than 5 percent of the Center's total net patient service revenue, it is a vital component. The lab currently performs 600 manometry tests per year. These tests measure the pressure (flow) along the gastrointestinal tract, which assists in the diagnosis of gastrointestinal disorders that cannot be diagnosed visually. The prevalence of disorders such as noncardiac chest pain, dysphasia, gastroesophageal reflux disease, and small bowel motility disorders make manometry testing beneficial to significant segments of the population.

Each test involves the insertion of catheters (probes) into a patient's gastrointestinal tract that relay data back to a computer work station for analysis. Two technologies are used in motility testing: water perfusion and solid-state. The Center currently has three water perfusion work stations dedicated to motility testing, each of which is used to perform roughly 200 tests per year.

Both water perfusion and solid-state technologies provide relatively reliable data for diagnosis. Furthermore, net reimbursement averages $250 per test regardless of technology, and the current per-test operating costs are identical: $150 for labor, $30 for medical supplies, and $15 for administrative supplies.

However, there are distinct differences between the two technologies, the most important of which is patient venue. Water perfusion technology requires the patient to spend one day as an inpatient, while solid-state technology can be done on an outpatient basis. Thus, each test that uses solid-state rather than water perfusion technology frees up one bed-day for other purposes. In general, the space freed up by new projects or technology is called "backfill space," so any beds made available for other purposes by replacing water perfusion with solid-state technology are called "backfill beds."

Although the Center is known for its state-of-the-art technology, its motility laboratory currently has some dated manometry equipment. The Center's medical director, Dr. Carl Forsyth, has made proposals in the past to update the equipment, but more pressing capital-investment needs within the Center have kept the proposals from being funded. However, one of the current work stations is becoming increasingly unreliable, which has inconvenienced patients and created backlogs. In addition, manometry demand has grown to the point where some patients are being referred to other providers to ensure timely testing. These factors have prompted the Center's administrative director, Edith Hargrove, to seek immediate approval for the acquisition of one new manometry system.

To begin the capital-expenditure request process, Edith is currently reviewing quotes from various manufacturers of manometry equipment. Her research on quality and cost has narrowed the field of competing manufacturers to one: Digestive Diagnostics, Inc. A water perfusion work station, which Edith favors, would cost $25,000, while the nine catheters needed to properly equip the work station would cost $500 each. The new generation of water perfusion systems, but **not** solid-state systems, has lower per-test supply costs: $15 for medical supplies and $10 for administrative supplies.

On the other hand, Dr. Forsyth believes that the Center should purchase a solid-state technology work station. Regardless of the technology purchased, the existing unreliable water perfusion work station would be "junked," as it is no longer capable of providing satisfactory service.

Edith, who is a clinically trained nurse, questions the clinical necessity of solid-state technology, especially in light of its higher cost. Although the cost of the work station is the same ($25,000), the cost of the catheters is substantially higher: $6,000 for each solid-state catheter versus $500 for each water perfusion catheter. Nine catheters are required for both technologies, so the total cost for catheters is $54,000 for solid-state technology versus only $4,500 for water perfusion technology. In addition, solid-state technology has higher operating (supply) costs than does the new water perfusion technology.

Dr. Forsyth agrees with the capital and operating cost estimates, but he argues that the higher cost of solid-state technology is justified for the following reasons:

1. Solid-state technology enables a technician to perform two tests in the time it takes to do one using water perfusion; rather than performing 200 tests per work station per year using water perfusion, 400 tests could be performed with solid-state. This would shorten patient wait time for appointments, decrease the current four-month backlog for motility testing, and potentially increase overall volume for the Center from 600 to 800 tests.
2. The current water perfusion technology requires close observation and correct body positioning during testing to ensure accurate data collection. As a result, each patient is kept in a hospital bed as an "observation" patient. Conversely, solid-state technology enables the tests to be performed on an outpatient basis. This point is of particular interest to the Hospital because under current operations every test using water perfusion is a bed-day that cannot be filled by a medical/surgical patient. Each bed-day by a "true" inpatient yields an average contribution margin of $520, whereas the bed-day contribution margin for a motility test patient is only $40.
3. Solid-state technology is quickly becoming the standard of care; not offering it would damage the Center's reputation.
4. Solid-state technology will enhance the teaching curriculum for residents and fellows and will provide additional opportunities for research funding.

To his credit, Dr. Forsyth is a respected physician with a reputation for providing the very best of patient care and at the same time remaining aware of his responsibilities to do so in the most cost-effective way possible. However, he has been criticized in the past for lobbying Hospital administrators for medical equipment that, in retrospect, could be labeled as being nothing more than "toys" for himself and his colleagues.

Edith listened to Dr. Forsyth's case for solid-state technology. She believes he makes some good points, especially in regard to the clinical efficiencies of solid-state technology. Still, in an environment where resources are limited and maintaining a positive bottom line is increasingly important, Edith continues to believe that the cost of the solid-state catheters is a financial burden the lab cannot afford, especially when reimbursement is the same regardless of the technology used.

The two technology proposals have been brought to the attention of the Hospital's chief operating officer, Belinda Brach, for resolution. Believing that a detailed financial analysis is the only rational basis for a decision, she has asked you, a recently hired financial analyst, to investigate the situation. Specifically, you have been asked to use capital-budgeting techniques to evaluate the two technologies and make a recommendation on which one to choose.

In addition, Belinda provided some much needed guidance. First, assume that the life of both technologies is five years and that it is unlikely that either the work stations or the catheters will have any salvage value after five years of use. Second, no good methodology is available to estimate the additional number of tests (more than 200) that might result from pent-up demand if solid-state technology is used. Volume might increase by 100 tests (to 300), but it could increase by as few as 50 or as many as 150. Third, it is difficult to say how many of the bed-days freed by the use of solid-state technology will actually be filled by medical/surgical patients. Again, without good data, she suggests you assume that 100 additional medical/surgical bed-days will result, but this number could be as low as 80 or as high as 175. Fourth, standard practice calls for all capital-budgeting analyses to assume a 3 percent inflation rate in both costs and reimbursements. Finally, the Hospital's corporate cost of capital is 10 percent, and it adds or subtracts 3 percentage points to account for differential risk.

Just as you were about to start the analysis, the phone rang; it was Belinda. She said it was likely that she could put her hands on some additional funding to buy a second system, but the amount will only be enough to buy a water perfusion system. When you asked Edith what the lab will do with the second current system, if it too should be replaced, she said the Hospital could sell it for about $10,000 because it is only three years old. Edith added, "You might as well crunch the numbers on the potential second system while you're at it."

Working Capital

COMMONWEALTH PHARMACEUTICALS
RECEIVABLES MANAGEMENT

27

KATHLEEN GROGAN received her PhD in pharmacology ten years ago from Boston University. While there, she became interested in the business side of drug distribution and hence stayed on for an extra 18 months to earn an MBA. After graduation, she went to work for Criser Corporation, a major drug manufacturer, where she managed the development of a new nonprescription anti-allergy drug. Although the drug passed all FDA (Food and Drug Administration) trials and was certified for general use, Criser simultaneously developed a similar drug that was cheaper to produce and equally effective in treating most, but not all, allergy symptoms. Thus, Criser decided not to proceed with production of the drug that Kathleen helped develop. However, Criser was willing to license production and distribution rights to another company. Kathleen thought that this might be a golden opportunity, so she quit her job with Criser to found her own company, Commonwealth Pharmaceuticals. The sole purpose of the new company is to obtain the license for, produce, and distribute the new drug, which Kathleen dubbed "SneezeRelief."

Kathleen is currently working on the business plan that she will present at a venture capital conference to be held in New York. The main purpose of the conference is to match entrepreneurs with venture capitalists who are interested in providing capital to fledgling firms. Kathleen has spent a lot of time thinking about how her proposed company's receivables should be managed; she is concerned about this issue because she knows of several small drug manufacturers that have gotten into serious financial difficulty because of poor receivables management.

Initially, Commonwealth Pharmaceuticals will sell directly and exclusively to four retail customers in the Northeast (Exhibit 27.1 provides the sales mix). If demand proves solid, the company will expand into other areas and wholesale channels. Sales are expected to be highly seasonal: Allergy drug sales are slow during the winter months, but they pick up dramatically in the spring when plant pollen levels reach a peak. Business falls off again in the summer, but it picks up in the fall when the ragweed season begins. Kathleen's sales forecasts for the first six months of operations are given in Exhibit 27.2. Assuming the fledgling company receives financing and begins operations, Kathleen's sales forecasts for the first six months of the second year are contained in Exhibit 27.3.

Kathleen does not plan to give discounts for early payment; discounts are not widely used in the industry. Based on preliminary discussions with the retail outlets (her customers), Kathleen forecasts the payment schedule shown in Exhibit 27.4. She does not foresee any problems with bad debt losses; the retailers to whom she plans to sell have been in business a long time. Furthermore, she plans to carefully screen her customers, and she believes that these two factors will eliminate such losses. On average, Kathleen believes that 20 percent of receivables will contribute to profits, so 80 percent of receivables represent cash costs. Furthermore, the First National Bank of New England has indicated that its receivables financing will cost 10 percent annually.

In spite of her optimism regarding bad debt losses, Kathleen is concerned about the company's potential level of receivables, and she wants to have a monitoring system in place that will allow her to quickly spot any adverse trends if they develop. Kathleen's total sales forecast for the first full year of operations is 800,000 packages. Each package, which will contain 12 tablets, will be priced at $5.

Kathleen would like you, an outside consultant, to develop the following first-year data for the venture capital conference:

1. The company's projected average collection period (ACP), also called days sales outstanding (DSO)

2. The company's projected average daily sales (Use a 360-day year.)
3. The company's projected average receivables level
4. The end-of-year balance sheet figures for accounts receivable and notes payable, assuming that notes payable are used to finance the investment in receivables
5. The projected annual dollar cost of carrying the receivables
6. The receivables level at the end of March and the end of June (Note that the receivables level forecasts, and all forecasts required by the following questions, should be based on these assumptions: (a) the sales mix in Exhibit 27.1 holds true, (b) the monthly sales forecasts given in Exhibit 27.2 are realized, and (c) the company's customers pay exactly as predicted in Exhibit 27.4.)
7. The company's forecasted average daily sales for the first three months of operations and for the entire half year
8. The implied ACP at the end of March and at the end of June
9. Aging schedules as of the end of March and the end of June

In addition, Kathleen remembered from her MBA program that uncollected balances schedules are superior to aging schedules in assessing receivables performance when sales are seasonal or cyclical. At the end of each quarter, the dollar amount of receivables remaining from each of the three month's sales is divided by that month's sales to obtain three receivables-to-sales ratios.

The uncollected balances schedule permits managers to remove the effects of seasonal and/or cyclical sales variation and to construct an accurate measure of receivables payment patterns. Thus, it provides financial managers with better aggregate information than such crude measures as the ACP or aging schedule. Because of their value, Kathleen also asked you to construct uncollected balances schedules as of the end of March and the end of June. Furthermore, she has asked you to use the uncollected balances schedule to forecast receivables levels at the ends of March and June of the second year of operations.

Kathleen anticipates that the venture capitalists will ask some questions concerning both the interpretation of the receivables data and the sensitivity of the results to the basic assumptions. Thus, be prepared to thoroughly discuss the results of your analysis.

EXHIBIT 27.1
Commonwealth Pharmaceuticals: Customer Sales Mix Forecast

Customer	Sales Mix
Large Retail Chain 1	40%
Large Retail Chain 2	35%
Regional Drug Store	17%
Small Grocery Chain	8%

EXHIBIT 27.2
Commonwealth Pharmaceuticals: Partial Sales Forecasts for Year 1

Month	Sales
January	$100,000
February	250,000
March	400,000
April	600,000
May	450,000
June	300,000

EXHIBIT 27.3
Commonwealth Pharmaceuticals: Partial Sales Forecasts for Year 2

Month	Sales
January	$200,000
February	350,000
March	500,000
April	700,000
May	550,000
June	350,000

Customer	0–30 days	30–60 days	60–90 days
Large Retail Chain 1	35%	50%	15%
Large Retail Chain 2	25%	40%	35%
Regional Drug Store	20%	35%	45%
Small Grocery Chain	30%	55%	15%

EXHIBIT 27.4 Commonwealth Pharmaceuticals: Receivables Collection Pattern Forecast

CLEAR LAKE HOSPITAL
INVENTORY MANAGEMENT

28

CLEAR LAKE HOSPITAL is a 230-bed, not-for-profit, acute care hospital located in Clear Lake, Iowa. The lake, for which the city and hospital are named, is dotted with vacation homes and is a major summer resort and fishing area. In addition, the city is the site of the 1959 small plane crash that killed rock and roll musicians Buddy Holly, Ritchie Valens, and J. P. "The Big Bopper" Richardson.

The hospital carries more than 10,000 different items of inventory that vary widely in price, order lead times, and stockout costs. (Stockout costs are the total costs that result from running out of stock of a particular inventory item, including higher costs of service caused by scheduling delays or emergency replenishments as well as the costs associated with negative outcomes and potential lawsuits.)

Clear Lake uses the ABC method of inventory classification, along with a variety of inventory-control methods, to manage its different inventory items. The ABC inventory classification system works in this way. Clear Lake maintains data on the average annual usage and unit cost of each inventory item, which typically is called a stock keeping unit (SKU). Then, the dollar usage (Average annual usage × Unit cost) is calculated for each SKU. Next, these amounts are converted into percentages of total dollar usage and the SKUs are arrayed from highest to lowest percentage. The SKUs are then divided into three groups (or classes), labeled A, B, and C, using the general guidance contained in Exhibit 28.1.

To better use the limited resources available for inventory management, the hospital's managers focus most of their attention on Class A items. The usage rates, stock positions, and delivery times for SKUs in this class are reviewed on a biweekly basis, with control and ordering system data adjusted as necessary. Class B items are reviewed every quarter, while Class C items are reviewed semiannually.

Even though this process has served Clear Lake well, Julio Ruiz, the hospital's newly hired chief financial officer, thinks the hospital is carrying excess inventories. He notes that Clear Lake has never come close to having a stockout, even when it has been running near 100 percent occupancy. Julio believes that a thorough review should be undertaken of all Class A items, and that it might be possible to increase inventory turnover by 25 percent, and hence lower inventory carrying costs, by trimming current stocks.

To convince Clear Lake's chief executive officer (CEO), Julio plans to perform a demonstration inventory analysis that focuses on the forms used by the surgical intensive care unit (SICU). Different forms are required for almost every aspect of SICU operations, including records of patient progress; requests for lab tests, blood, and medications; nurse and physician notes; and transfer/discharge instructions. Exhibit 28.2 contains inventory usage and cost data on the SICU's 25 forms. To begin his demonstration analysis, Julio plans to conduct a new ABC analysis on the SICU's inventory.

As part of its commitment to supporting the local economy, Clear Lake currently uses a single, local source for all of the SICU's forms: Atwood Printing and Office Supplies (Supplier A). Supplier A requires a $25 set-up fee on each order, in addition to the cost per unit. Clear Lake is considering using a national supplier, Bateman Medical Office Products (Supplier B), that charges no set-up fee but does charge $50 to cover postage and handling. Supplier B takes three days to deliver the forms, versus only one day delivery offered by Supplier A. Processing each order will cost the hospital another $25, regardless of which supplier is used. Thus, the total order cost is $50 for Supplier A and $75 for Supplier B.

Julio's ultimate goal is to use economic ordering quantity (EOQ) concepts to select the supplier for all forms used by the SICU. His primary areas of concern are (1) the number of orders placed each year, (2) reorder points (in units), and (3) total inventory costs. As part of the demonstration analysis, Julio will focus on the form used to order blood products from the hospital's blood bank (SKU number 53104 in Exhibit 28.2). The data associated with Suppliers A and B, as well as inventory carrying costs and other data, are summarized in Exhibit 28.3.

In addition to an analysis without safety stocks, Julio is also concerned about the impact of safety stocks on the decision. Clear Lake currently carries a safety stock of two units of SKU 53104 to protect itself against stockouts as a result of delivery delays and/or an increase in the usage rate. When asked how that amount was calculated, the manager of the SICU stated that she did not know, but they had always done it that way. However, if the hospital decides to switch to Supplier B, she said it seems logical to increase the safety stock to six units to reflect Supplier B's three-times-as-long lead time. Of particular interest are the impact of safety stocks on inventory costs, the safety margins that such stocks provide against higher-than-expected usage and shipping delays, and whether or not the current lead time for Supplier A and the estimate for Supplier B make any sense.

Also, Julio has heard a rumor that Supplier B is about to offer a 10 percent discount if the entire year's demand (92 units) is ordered at once. He wants to know the impact of this discount on the decision about which supplier to use. Also, it would be good to know how high a discount must be to make Supplier B less costly than Supplier A.

Furthermore, Julio knows it is unlikely that the forms will be ordered exactly as prescribed by the EOQ model, so he would like to know the impact of ordering variations on total inventory costs. Finally, Julio knows that Clear Lake's CEO has expressed some doubt about the value of the EOQ model in making real-world inventory decisions. "If I'm right in my concerns," he asked, "what other inventory control methods are available to us?"

Place yourself in Julio's shoes and see if you can conduct the demonstration analysis that he has in mind.

Classification	Inventory Value	Inventory Amount
A	60–70%	10–20%
B	20–30%	30–40%
C	10–20%	50–60%

EXHIBIT 28.1
ABC Classification Guidance

EXHIBIT 28.2
Clear Lake Hospital: Form Inventory Data for the Surgical Intensive Care Unit

SKU Number	Unit Size	Supplier A Unit Cost	Units Used Annually
50071	25	$31	3
50083	25	16	4
50084	50	18	14
50091	250	86	28
50100	25	22	4
50102	250	793	3
50122	250	196	2
50129	250	177	3
50131	100	122	5
50132	100	98	5
50138	100	26	9
50139	50	21	10
50170	100	8	83
50172	100	44	4
50174	500	62	8
50193	25	2	66
50194	100	122	2
50206	250	11	279
50472	100	192	2
50475	125	551	4
50694	100	18	10
51060	100	102	6
53006	50	17	4
53104	50	66	92
57134	100	16	5

EXHIBIT 28.3
Clear Lake Hospital Cost and Usage Data: Blood Product Ordering Form (SKU 53104)

Expected annual usage	92 units
Cost per unit:	
Supplier A	$66
Supplier B	$60
Inventory carrying costs:	
Depreciation	0.0%
Storage and handling	17.1
Interest expense	6.6
Property taxes	0.4
Insurance	0.9
Total carrying costs	25.0%
Inventory ordering costs:	
Supplier A	$50
Supplier B	$75
Current safety stocks:	
Supplier A	2 units
Supplier B (estimate)	6 units
Delivery times:	
Supplier A	1 day
Supplier B	3 days

Other Topics

RIVERVIEW COMMUNITY HOSPITAL (B)

29

FINANCIAL FORECASTING

RIVERVIEW COMMUNITY HOSPITAL is a 210-bed, not-for-profit, acute care hospital with a long-standing reputation for quality service to a growing community. Riverview competes with three other hospitals in its metropolitan statistical area—two not-for-profit and one for-profit. Riverview is the smallest of the four but has traditionally been ranked highest in patient satisfaction surveys. For a more complete description of the hospital, along with its 2005–2009 financial statements, see Case 1: Riverview Community Hospital (A).

As the newly hired special assistant to the CEO, you have completed the financial and operating analyses (Case 1) assigned by your boss, Melissa Randolph. In fact, your presentation to the board of trustees went so well that Melissa asked you to present the hospital's preliminary five-year financial plan at the next board meeting. To aid in the planning process, she provided the following information:

1. Given your knowledge of the historical situation for Riverview, current trends in the healthcare industry, and the competitive situation facing hospitals today, use your own best judgment to create the hospital's financial plan. Make any assumptions you believe to be necessary to create the plan, including assumptions about inpatient and outpatient volume growth, capacity constraints, reimbursement patterns, hospital staffing patterns, input cost inflation, and so on. Be

sure to completely document your assumptions in the report. **The quality of your financial plan will be judged as much (or more so) on the validity of your assumptions as on the mechanics of the forecasting process.** (You have limited specific information about Riverview, so use your general knowledge about trends in the hospital industry to make the forecasts.)

2. The emphasis should be on the forecast for the first year (2010), but you should also create rough income statements, balance sheets, and statements of cash flows for the coming five years, including key financial ratios.

3. The five primary methods for forecasting income statement items and balance sheet accounts are (a) percentage of sales (in which a constant growth rate is applied), (b) simple linear regression, (c) curvilinear regression, (d) multiple regression, and (e) specific item forecasting. You may need to use several of these methods in your forecast. (Hint: Do not forget that spreadsheets have a regression capability.)

4. Use the financial analysis from Case 1 to help with the forecast if this case is assigned. Those areas where hospital performance has been poor should be improved, and your forecasts should reflect anticipated operational improvements where applicable.

5. Do not get so involved in the mechanics of the forecasting process that you forget to apply common sense to your forecasts. Think about what has happened in the past and what is likely to happen in the future in regard to utilization, prices, costs, and asset requirements. If the forecast does not make sense, modify it until it does. For example, a blind application of statistical forecasting techniques might lead to a forecast containing five years of net operating losses. Regardless of statistical "fit," such a forecast makes no sense because any hospital, if it expects to survive, will have to take actions to change either utilization or cost trends to ensure positive operating results. Thus,

the "blindly" forecasted values do not represent what is likely to happen in the future, even though they might be a perfect reflection of historical trends. Also, a forecast that is wildly optimistic probably needs to be modified because payers will react negatively if hospital profits rise dramatically.

In closing, Melissa gave you her view of a good financial plan: "First and foremost, the plan should consist of pro forma financial statements along with a table that summarizes the amount of financing generated internally and any external financing requirements. Second, key financial ratios should be calculated, and the hospital's expected future financial condition should be assessed, with special emphasis on changes from the hospital's current condition. Third, make sure that your forecasted financial statements are consistent with one another. The last special assistant could not figure out that some balance sheet accounts—equity (fund) capital and accumulated depreciation—are tied to income statement items, so he did not last very long. Finally, make all your assumptions clear, and be prepared to answer questions from the board concerning the impact of changes in your assumptions on the financial plan."

COPPERLINE HEALTHCARE

CAPITATION AND RISK SHARING

30

COPPERLINE MEMORIAL HOSPITAL is a community hospital in Green Bay, Wisconsin. Recently, the hospital and its affiliated physicians formed Copperline Healthcare, a physician hospital organization (the PHO). The PHO is close to signing its first contract to provide exclusive local healthcare services to enrollees in BadgerCare (the Plan), the local Blue Cross Blue Shield of Wisconsin HMO. For the past several years, the Plan has contracted with a different Green Bay PHO, but financial difficulties at that organization have prompted the Plan to consider Copperline Healthcare as an alternative. In the proposed contract, the PHO will assume full risk for patient utilization. In fact, the proposal calls for the PHO to receive a fixed premium of $200 per member per month from the Plan, which it then can allocate to each provider component in any way it deems best using any reimbursement method it chooses.

The PHO's executive director, Dr. George O'Donnell, a cardiologist and recent graduate of the University of Wisconsin's Nonresident Program in Administrative Medicine, is evaluating the Plan's proposal. To help do this, Dr. O'Donnell hired a consulting firm that specializes in PHO contracting.

The first task of the consulting firm was to review the PHO's current medical panel and estimate the number of physicians, by specialty, required to support the Plan's patient population of 50,000, assuming aggressive utilization management. The results in Exhibit 30.1 show that the PHO's medical panel currently consists of 249 physicians, while the number of physicians required to support the Plan's patient population is only 59. Note, however, that the PHO physicians serve patients other than those in the Plan, so the total number of physicians required to treat all of the PHO's patients far exceeds the 59 shown in the right column of the table.

The second task of the consulting firm was to analyze the PHO physicians' current practice patterns. Clearly, utilization, and hence cost, is driven by the PHO's physicians and variation in practice patterns is costly to the PHO. Results of the analysis show significant variation in practice patterns, both in the physicians' offices and in the hospital. For example, Exhibit 30.2 contains summary data on hospital costs by physician for three common diagnosis-related groups (DRGs). Consider DRG 127 (heart failure). The physician with the lowest hospital costs averaged $4,271 in costs per patient, the highest cost physician averaged $7,394, and the average cost for all physicians was $5,319. The consulting firm commented that reducing this variation is important because the PHO is at full risk for patient utilization.

The third task of the consulting firm was to recommend an appropriate allocation of the premium dollars to each category of provider. More specifically, the contract calls for the PHO to receive $200 per member per month, for a total annual revenue of $200 × 50,000 members × 12 months = $120 million. To reduce potential conflicts about how to divide the $120 million among providers, the consulting firm proposed a "status quo" allocation that would maintain the current revenue distribution percentages shown in Exhibit 30.3.

The final task of the consulting firm was to recommend provider reimbursement methodologies that create appropriate incentives. In the contract, the PHO assumes full risk for patient utilization, so the consulting firm recommended that all component providers be capitated to align cost minimization incentives across the entire PHO. Furthermore, capitation of all providers eliminates the need for risk pools, a risk sharing arrangement that the PHO has never used.

In addition to the consulting firm's report, Dr. O'Donnell decided to ask the new PHO operations committee for a short report on the current status of the major PHO providers. He was provided with the following information.

Copperline Memorial Hospital

Historically, the profitability of Copperline Memorial Hospital has been roughly in line with the industry. Last year, when the hospital received about 75 percent of charges, on average, it achieved an operating margin of about 3 percent. However, hospital managers are concerned about its profitability if the Plan's proposal is accepted. The managers believe that the full risk contract requires extraordinary efforts to control costs and that the most effective way to do so is to create a subpanel of physicians for participation in the capitation contract. When asked how the subpanel should be chosen, their reply was to choose physicians who could do the best job of containing hospital costs.

Primary Care Physicians

Many of the primary care physicians are dissatisfied. On average, primary care physicians receive only about 60 percent of charges, and they are concerned they could be penalized by accepting utilization risk for the Plan's enrollees. Primary care physicians know they are paid less and believe they have to work much harder than the specialists. Furthermore, primary care physicians believe the specialists supplement their own incomes by overusing in-office tests and procedures. Some primary care physicians are even talking about dropping out of the PHO, forming their own contracting group, and taking the whole capitation payment from the Plan and contracting themselves for specialist and hospital services.

Specialist Care Physicians

The specialists believe that the primary care physicians refer too many patients to them. The specialists do not mind the referrals as long as their reimbursement is based on charges because, on average, they receive 90 percent of charges. However, if they are capitated, the specialists want the primary care physicians to handle more of the minor patient problems themselves. Also, whenever the subject of subpanels is raised, many of the specialists become incensed. "After all," they say, "the whole idea behind the PHO is to protect the specialists." Both sets of physicians—primary care and specialists—agree that the hospital is hopelessly inefficient. Said one specialist, "no matter how much revenue the hospital receives, they still seem to barely make a profit."

To respond to the Plan's proposal, Dr. O'Donnell and the PHO's executive committee must decide whether to accept the recommendations of the consulting firm. More specifically, these questions must be addressed:

1. What proportion of the expected $200 per member per month capitation payment from the Plan should be allocated to each component (i.e., hospital, primary care physicians, specialists, and other providers)?
2. Are risk pools necessary? If so, what risk pools or other incentives should be put in place to help control utilization?
3. What payment method should be used for each provider? Should all providers be capitated, should any be capitated, or should some combination of methods be used?
4. Should all of the PHO physicians participate in the contract, or should subpanels be formed? If subpanels are formed, how should they be constituted?
5. What other actions must the PHO undertake to successfully manage this full-risk contract?

Assume that you have been hired to advise Dr. O'Donnell and the executive committee of Copperline Healthcare regarding its plan to address these challenges. At a minimum, your report should address all of the questions listed above as well as the concerns raised by the physicians and the hospital. Furthermore, the report must provide specific recommendations on how to implement these changes because the report will form the basis for an implementation plan if the contract is accepted. A general discussion about premium allocation, reimbursement methodologies, risk pools, subpanels, and so on, is not sufficient.

EXHIBIT 30.1
Copperline Healthcare: Physician PHO Members and Estimated Needs for 50,000 Enrollees

Specialty	Number in PHO	Estimated Need per 50,000 Enrollees
General medicine	42	20.9
Pediatrics	15	4.1
Total primary care	57	25.0
Anesthesiology	9	2.5
Cardiology	12	1.4
Emergency medicine	10	2.5
General surgery	13	2.7
Neurosurgery	3	0.3
Obstetrics/gynecology	27	5.4
Orthopedics	11	2.5
Psychiatry	19	1.9
Radiology	8	3.0
Thoracic surgery	0	0.4
Urology	5	1.3
Other specialties	75	10.1
Total specialists	192	34.0
Grand total	249	59.0

EXHIBIT 30.2
Hospital Costs for Three Common DRGs by Physician

DRG		Minimum	Average	Maximum
98:	Bronchitis/Asthma	$ 2,872	$ 4,018	$ 4,638
127:	Heart failure	4,271	5,319	7,394
373:	Vaginal delivery without complications	6,498	7,568	8,015

DRG: diagnosis-related group
Note: This table is based on historical costs related to the old severity-unadjusted DRGs. In the future, the cost data will be related to the new severity-adjusted MS-DRGs.

EXHIBIT 30.3
Proposed Allocation of Premium Dollars

PHO administration/overhead	13%
Paid to within-system physicians	
Primary care	10
Specialists	18
Ancillary services	5
Administration/profit	1
Paid to within-system hospital	38
Paid for prescription drugs	10
Paid to out-of-system providers	5
Total premium dollar	100%

Ethics
Mini-Cases

TRIGON BLUE CROSS/ BLUE SHIELD
COPAYMENTS

WHEN MOST PEOPLE are told they owe a coinsurance payment on a medical bill, they simply grimace and write a check; but not Gerald Haeckel, a retiree from Richmond, Virginia. He wanted proof that he was not paying more than the 20 percent portion that his health insurance policy required. When his insurer, Trigon Blue Cross/Blue Shield, balked, the retiree besieged state and federal officials with demands for an investigation.

Gerald's problem with insurer–provider negotiated discounts began when he became confused by a statement sent by Trigon Blue Cross/Blue Shield for his wife's lumpectomy, which is an outpatient surgery to remove a tiny breast tumor. Trigon's patient benefits statement indicated that the surgery had cost $950, that Trigon paid 80 percent or $760, and that Gerald owed a 20 percent copayment of $190. But then Gerald received a statement of charges and allowances from the surgery center indicating that Trigon's share of the bill had been more than halved to $374 because of a "contractual adjustment." Gerald assumed that a mistake was made in the surgery center's statement because if it were correct his $190 copayment would exceed a third of the actual cost, instead of the 20 percent called for in his healthcare policy's patient responsibility section.

Gerald's scrutiny of the $950 surgery bill led to a surprising discovery. Although insurance companies frequently complain about being duped by fraudulent policyholders and providers, Trigon and dozens of other health insurers and managed care companies stand accused of a scheme to siphon off millions of dollars from their policyholders. How does the alleged scheme work?

For surgery priced at $1,000, the typical plan might call for the insurer to pay 80 percent or $800, which leaves the patient with a $200 copayment. But if the insurer has negotiated a 50 percent discount from the provider and does not pass any of the savings on to its policyholders, the patient's $200 copayment becomes 40 percent of the $500 actual bill, and the insurer's portion drops to only $300.

Trigon's responses to Gerald's queries stirred up more questions than answers. Norwood H. Davis, Trigon's chief executive officer at the time, assured Gerald that he did indeed owe the $190 and added that the details of Trigon's provider contracts were "proprietary." In another letter, Norwood made a distinction between Trigon actually paying its $760 share of the bill and "discharging" it. Norwood added that although Trigon might try to persuade a provider to accept less than its $760 portion of the bill, a policyholder was free to do the same thing regarding the copayment. Gerald, who by that point was livid, replied, "suggesting that an individual policyholder negotiate with a provider for price concessions borders on the insulting!" and threatened to take the matter up with state regulators.

At a time when consumers are expected to take more responsibility for their own healthcare, undisclosed discounts raise questions about the accuracy and honesty of information provided by insurers, providers, and employers. Indeed, providers often are contractually prohibited from disclosing discounts. The insurance industry argues that hiding discounts is not widespread and the Chicago-based Blue Cross and Blue Shield Association notes that no court has ruled for plaintiffs in a discounts-related case. It adds that none of its affiliates that settled such cases admitted to wrongdoing. Furthermore, Blue Cross and Blue Shield executives argue that the discounts benefit policyholders by reducing premiums. In some situations, they add, employers who share in the savings ask that discounts not be disclosed to their own employees. "We're not lining our pockets with anything because there is nothing to line our pockets with," said Joel Gimpel, a Blue Cross and Blue Shield Association attorney.

What do you think about the copayment problem? Does this case present an ethical issue? If so, to which party (or parties)? If you could act as the ultimate authority in this situation, what would you do?

DEAL OF A LIFETIME
CORPORATE-OWNED LIFE INSURANCE

2

So what is new in the life insurance game? The answer is corporate ownership of life insurance policies on employees. Wal-Mart has been spending about $1 billion a year in premium payments to buy about $20 billion of life insurance coverage for 325,000 of its employees. Other big-name firms, such as Winn-Dixie, AT&T, Disney, GTE, Nestlé, and Procter & Gamble have been doing the same thing. Some (or even many) for-profit healthcare companies are probably doing the same thing, but no data are available to confirm this suspicion.

The product being bought by these companies is called corporate-owned life insurance (COLI), which is almost unknown outside of the insurance world. In fact, insurers typically call COLI "janitors' insurance" to distinguish it from the life insurance that companies often take out on key executives to help offset their loss to the company from premature death and from corporate-provided life insurance that is part of a business's managerial fringe-benefit program. In fact, one corporate executive at Winn-Dixie was accused of calling COLI "dead peasants' insurance" in an interoffice memo. Needless to say, Winn-Dixie would not comment on the accusation.

Here is an overview of how COLI works:

1. A company takes out, say, a $100,000 life insurance policy on one of its lower-level employees. The employee may or may not have to agree to the policy, depending on the state. If it is necessary to

get employee approval, the company may offer to pay a small amount—say, $5,000—to the family if the individual dies while an employee of the firm or $1,000 if the individual has left the firm. This payment to the employee's family costs the employee nothing, so finding willing participants is not hard when worker approval is required.

2. To pay for the policy, the company borrows the entire premium from the insurance company that issues the policy. Usually, the policies are single-premium policies, so only one up-front payment is made. The company also borrows the money needed to make the interest payments on the loan, so no cash would flow from the employee's company to the insurance company while the policy is in force.

3. The company's bottom line is helped in two ways. First, increases in the paid-in cash value of the policy are reported as profits. Second, the company receives a tax-free death benefit when the employee dies, even if he or she has long ago left the company.

4. The company uses the tax-free death benefit to pay off the policy loan and to make the payment to the family, if one was promised, and then pockets the difference.

Most companies claim they use the money received from insurance benefits to pay for various employee and retiree benefit programs. However, this is difficult to verify, and there is no requirement to do so. Furthermore, each dollar from COLI that is used for employee and retiree benefits frees another dollar to be used for executive compensation and perquisites.

What do you think about the concept of "dead peasants' insurance"? Does this case present an ethical issue? If so, to which party (or parties)? If you could act as the ultimate authority in this situation, what would you do?

BAYVIEW SURGERY CENTER

3

PRICING/BILLING OF SURGICAL SERVICES

JOYCE GRIFFIN is an accountant who is also an avid tennis player. One fall afternoon, after an inspiring win at the tennis club, she noticed a sharp pain in her knee. The diagnosis was a torn tendon, which could be easily corrected by arthroscopic surgery. After consultation with an orthopedic surgeon whom she knew from the club, Joyce asked the physician to schedule the surgery for the following week at Bayview Surgery Center (the Center), a local outpatient surgery center.

Being an accountant and detail minded, Joyce called the Center as soon as the surgery was scheduled to provide the required insurance information and to ascertain the amount of the charge. The patient accounts clerk at the Center quoted a charge of $1,500 for the surgery and told Joyce to bring a check for $300 the day of the surgery to cover the 20 percent copayment called for by her health insurance policy. Joyce paid the $300, and, fortunately, the surgery was a resounding success. In fact, Joyce was extremely pleased with the medical care provided both by the Center and the surgeon.

The problems began the following week when Joyce received a copy of the bill that was submitted to her insurance company. Her eyes almost popped out when she read the total, $2,657, which should have required a copayment of $531. Equally strange was that the insurance claim form showed no sign of her $300 copayment; the "Amount Paid" space had a zero. Confused by the inconsistencies between what she had been told earlier and the claims form, she confronted the Center's business manager for an explanation. The best answer she could get was, "This is just the way we do it. Everybody does it this way."

There are two ways of looking at this dual pricing of services. First, perhaps the Center is trying to give the patients—the "little guys"—a break; we might call this the "Robin Hood theory" of billing. Second, the Center might be trying to increase business by quoting a lower price to patients, and hence charging a lower copayment, but making up for the lower copayment by charging the insurance company more.

Neither of these possible explanations were satisfying to Joyce, so she informed her insurance company and asked them what they planned to do about the Center's pricing inconsistencies. But much to her shock and disappointment, her insurance company did not seem to care. Even worse, the letter she received contained these sentences: "We don't print money; we handle money. Do not worry about us overpaying for services because you, the consumer, through your employer, are ultimately paying for this."

What do you think about quoting one price for patients and another for insurers? Does this case present an ethical issue? If so, to which party (or parties)? If you could act as the ultimate authority in this situation, what would you do?

JEFFERSON GENERAL HOSPITAL

4

MERGERS, ACQUISITIONS, AND AGENCY

MARK MILLER, chief executive officer (CEO) of Jefferson General Hospital, has some tough decisions to make in the future. Jefferson General is a stand-alone, not-for-profit hospital that has a long and proud tradition of serving the community in which it operates. It was founded in the midst of the great depression as Jefferson County Hospital and remained under public control for more than 50 years. Then, in 1986, after years of losses, the county decided that it could no longer afford to operate the hospital, and it subsequently converted the hospital from a public to a private entity. At that time, Mark was brought in as the CEO. After a shaky start, he was able to turn the hospital into a moneymaker. Still, he was aware of the hospital's roots, and he made sure that the hospital continued its original mission of providing healthcare services to the needy, regardless of their ability to pay.

Jefferson General is the smallest of the three hospitals that serve Jefferson and surrounding counties; the other two are St. Vincent's Hospital and Northwest Regional Medical Center. St. Vincent's has religious roots, but it is now operated as a not-for-profit, nonsectarian hospital. Northwest Regional is owned and operated by a large for-profit chain. The combined capacity of the three hospitals is more than 950 beds, but none of the three operates above 60 percent occupancy. Furthermore, managed care is starting to take hold locally, and hospital utilization trends indicate that the service area will need only 600 beds as utilization rates and the length of inpatient stays are squeezed down.

The most logical solution to the county's changing healthcare market conditions is a merger between two of the three hospitals, and Jefferson General is the hospital most likely to be acquired. Mark has been approached by the CEOs of both St. Vincent's and Northwest Regional concerning his interest in a merger. Although it is too early to speculate on the exact terms that might result if a merger takes place, past mergers in the region provide some insights into what might happen to Mark should a merger occur.

If the hospital is acquired by St. Vincent's, Mark will likely continue as CEO of the hospital and earn about the same compensation as he currently receives. However, he may lose much of his autonomy and authority because he will have to report to the system CEO, who most likely will be the current CEO of St. Vincent's. If the hospital is acquired by Northwest Regional, Mark will probably relocate to a CEO position at some other not-for-profit hospital because the for-profit chain usually brings in its own management team when it makes an acquisition. But Mark will not go away empty handed. He will likely receive a large "golden parachute" as a result of his job loss, which might include lucrative stock options, a lump sum payment, and a consulting contract. The aggregate amount of such payments could easily be worth many times his current annual salary.

Although the ultimate decision regarding the fate of Jefferson General rests in the hands of its board of trustees, the members of the board were chosen more on the basis of their community ties than on their business acumen. Thus, all those involved are aware that Mark's recommendations regarding the hospital's future will carry a great deal of weight in the final decision.

What do you think about the dilemma facing Mark Miller? Does this case present an ethical issue? If so, to which party (or parties)? If you could act as the ultimate authority in this situation, what would you do?

FRONT STREET HOSPITAL

UNINSURED CHARGES AND COLLECTIONS

5

WHO IS RICHARD "Dickie" Scruggs, and what does he have to do with hospital finance? You may not be familiar with the name, but you will undoubtedly read about his work and its influence on how uninsured patients are billed and the manner in which the bills are collected. You see, Dickie Scruggs runs a law firm in Pascagoula, Mississippi, that made huge amounts of money out of multibillion-dollar settlements from asbestos and tobacco companies. Now, his law firm is taking on the not-for-profit hospital industry. (To find out about his more recent activities, both good and bad, do a Wikipedia search on Dickie Scruggs.)

His firm has filed more than 70 lawsuits in federal courts against not-for-profit hospitals, alleging that the hospitals routinely overcharge self-pay patients, hound them with aggressive collection tactics, and fail to provide adequate charity care in violation of their tax-exempt status. In a number of the lawsuits, the American Hospital Association (AHA) is named as a coconspirator and defendant. Needless to say, the AHA has called the lawsuits "baseless" and a diversion of resources that could otherwise be used for community healthcare.

The heart of the lawsuits revolves around two issues. First, the fact that patients who are least able to pay are generally charged the most. It is common practice to bill self-pay patients at full charges, whereas most every other payer is paying less than full charges, often substantially less. For example, consider the case of Jane Adams, age

22 and uninsured, who recently spent two days in not-for-profit Front Street Hospital for an appendectomy procedure. Her hospital bill was $14,000, and doctor's fees added another $5,000. It turns out that if a local HMO had insured Jane, the hospital bill would have been about $2,500. Medicaid would have paid about $5,000, and Medicare would have paid about $7,800 for the same procedure. "Why do I get stuck with the whole bill?" asked Jane. "An uninsured person has a lot less money than insurance companies or government agencies."

Unfortunately, Jane stumbled onto a troubling fact of hospital finance: Most hospitals set official "charges" for their services but then agree to discount those charges for third-party payers. As a result, almost no one but the uninsured ever pays "official" charges. In some ways, hospital charges are like hotel "rack rates," which are posted prices that everybody knows nobody pays. But the hospital industry is different, because uninsured patients traditionally have been billed the equivalent of rack rates.

The second element of the lawsuits revolves around collection tactics. Although hospitals collect less than 5 percent of billings from indigent patients, many hospitals are aggressive in their collection tactics. A press release announcing the lawsuits said that hospitals engage in business methods calculated to defeat the rights of uninsured patients. According to Scruggs, if and when the uninsured patient can't pay, not-for-profit hospitals often intimidate and harass uninsured patients through "goon-like and predatory collection tactics that frequently scar the patient for life, including the trauma of personal bankruptcy."

To illustrate, consider the case of Marlin Bushman, who was arrested, handcuffed, and taken to jail for missing a court hearing about a $579 Front Street bill. This collection tactic, known as "body attachment," has been abandoned by most other creditors. Said one observer, "The concept of debtor's prison as we understand it from Dickens' time is alive and well in the hospital industry." Another favorite strong-arm tactic is to place a lien on the patient's house. For example, Front Street placed a $3,600 lien on the house of Ben Pickett for a $3,000 unpaid hospital bill. Furthermore, a threat was made to foreclose, and hence force Ben to sell the house, if the debt was not paid within 90 days. The interest on the debt was pegged at 12 percent, which means that Ben will never be able to pay it off because the interest is accruing faster than his ability to make payments.

The worst part of these billing and collection tactics, according to Scruggs, is that these policies are deliberately put in place to discourage the indigent from seeking healthcare services. By discouraging uninsured patients from seeking healthcare, not-for-profit hospitals are avoiding their obligation to provide charitable services as required by their not-for-profit status.

What do you think about the billing and collection policies of not-for-profit hospitals related to the uninsured? Does this case present an ethical issue? If so, to which party (or parties)? If you could act as the ultimate authority in this situation, what would you do?

WESTWOOD IMAGING CENTERS
PAYMENT FOR REFERRALS

6

MEDICAL IMAGING IS one of healthcare's fastest-growing sectors, so most everyone wants to get in on the action, including physicians. To illustrate, imaging costs are Medicare's fastest-growing service item. In recent years, they rose at three times the rate of other medical services, and the total spent on imaging services exceeded $100 billion in 2008. One reason for this rapid increase is the ability of imaging to detect conditions that previously required diagnostic surgery for detection. But another reason could be the financial incentives that make some doctors order more scans than are medically necessary.

At a recent meeting of cardiologists, neurologists, and oncologists, Westwood Imaging Centers told doctors how they could get in on the boom. The deal works like this:

- Doctors send patients to Westwood for imaging services, and Westwood charges the referring physician a flat rate per scan.
- Then, the physician bills the third-party payer for the scan at the going rate. For example, Westwood charges physicians $375 for an MRI scan, while the average reimbursement for the scan is estimated at about $700. After deducting about $90 per scan for interpretation and administrative costs (mostly billing and collections), the profit per scan comes in at about $235 per referral.

A group practice that refers ten patients a day pockets about $600,000 annually under this plan. For more expensive PET scans, the same volume produces an annual profit for the referring group of more than $2 million. For the most part, the third-party payers are unaware of the deal, assuming that the scans are conducted in the doctor's office.

But wait a minute, aren't such arrangements against the law? After all, federal antikickback laws prohibit providers such as Westwood from paying doctors for referrals when Medicare or Medicaid patients are involved. These laws also extend to other types of patients under 36 state statutes. The Westwood plan also raises the issue of "self-referral," which occurs when physicians refer patients to businesses in which they or relatives have a financial interest. When these prohibitions are considered, isn't the Westwood proposal illegal?

It turns out that there are exceptions to the antikickback and self-referral laws. One exception is that it is all right to self-refer when the services are done in the physician's office. For example, it is legal to order an electrocardiogram for a patient and then perform the procedure in the doctor's office. Clearly, the Westwood proposal does not meet the exception because it is done at Westwood's imaging center.

Westwood's solution to the legality issue is to characterize the scan not as a referral but rather as a "per use, non-recurring lease agreement." In other words, when the scan is performed, the equipment and the space around it are "owned" by the referring physician, and hence the scan qualifies as a procedure done in the doctor's office. Some imaging companies are using a slightly different approach. Instead of paying a charge for each scan, the physician (or group) books a set number of hours per week on a scanner, which they must pay even if they don't send enough patients to use all the time booked. This arrangement adds risk to the physician but supposedly is more resistant to antikickback laws.

Does anyone get hurt by such deals? Virtually all research done in this area indicates that utilization increases when doctors have a financial stake in providing imaging services. For example, one New York neurology practice with a lease deal ordered almost 50 percent more scans than did similar practices without such deals. It is hard to believe that the increased cost to insurers is medically justified, so the third-party payers (and ultimately the purchasers of health insurance) end up paying more than is necessary.

What do you think about Westwood's proposal to provide physicians with "leased" diagnostic equipment? Does this case present an ethical issue? If so, to which party (or parties)? If you could act as the ultimate authority in this situation, what would you do?

About the Author

LOUIS C. GAPENSKI, PhD, is a professor in both health services administration and finance at the University of Florida. He is the author or coauthor of more than 20 textbooks on corporate and healthcare finance. Dr. Gapenski's books are used worldwide, with Canadian and international editions as well as translations into Bulgarian, Chinese, French, Indonesian, Italian, Polish, Portuguese, Russian, and Spanish. In addition, he has published more than 40 journal articles related to corporate and healthcare finance.

Dr. Gapenski is an active member of the Association of University Programs in Health Administration, the American College of Healthcare Executives, and the Healthcare Financial Management Association. He has acted as academic advisor, chaired sessions, and presented papers at numerous national meetings. Additionally, Dr. Gapenski has been an editorial board member and reviewer for 12 academic and professional journals.

About the Contributor

GEORGE H. PINK, PhD, is a professor in the Department of Health Policy and Administration, School of Public Health at the University of North Carolina at Chapel Hill and is a Senior Research Fellow at the Cecil G. Sheps Center for Health Services Research at the University of North Carolina at Chapel Hill. Prior to receiving a doctorate in corporate finance, he spent ten years in health services management, planning, and consulting.

Dr. Pink teaches courses in healthcare finance and is involved in several large research projects, including studies of hospital financial performance. In the past 20 years, he has served on boards and committees of more than 100 hospitals and other healthcare organizations. He has written more than 60 peer-reviewed articles and has made more than 200 academic presentations in ten countries.